107 Powerful Breast Cancer Meal and Juice Recipes:

Fight Breast Cancer by Using Natural Vitamin-Rich Foods

By

Joe Correa CSN

COPYRIGHT

This publication is designed to provide accurate and authoritative information in regard to the subject matter covered. It is sold with the understanding that neither the author nor the publisher is engaged in rendering medical advice. If medical advice or assistance is needed, consult with a doctor. This book is considered a guide and should not be used in any way detrimental to your health. Consult with a physician before starting this nutritional plan to make sure it's right for you.

ACKNOWLEDGEMENTS

This book is dedicated to my friends and family that have had mild or serious illnesses so that you may find a solution and make the necessary changes in your life.

107 Powerful Breast Cancer Meal and Juice Recipes:

Fight Breast Cancer by Using Natural Vitamin-Rich Foods

By

Joe Correa CSN

CONTENTS

Copyright

Acknowledgements

About The Author

Introduction

107 Powerful Breast Cancer Meal and Juice Recipes: Fight Breast Cancer by Using Natural Vitamin-Rich Foods

Additional Titles from This Author

ABOUT THE AUTHOR

After years of Research, I honestly believe in the positive effects that proper nutrition can have over the body and mind. My knowledge and experience has helped me live healthier throughout the years and which I have shared with family and friends. The more you know about eating and drinking healthier, the sooner you will want to change your life and eating habits.

Nutrition is a key part in the process of being healthy and living longer so get started today. The first step is the most important and the most significant.

INTRODUCTION

107 Powerful Breast Cancer Meal and Juice Recipes: Fight Breast Cancer by Using Natural Vitamin-Rich Foods

By Joe Correa CSN

Prevent breast cancer if possible and if you already have breast cancer take the necessary steps to give your body the power to find a way to heal through food. Trust your body and your instincts. What you eat and drink will determine just how equipped your body is to recover. Give it junk food and expect no less. Give it clean, raw, and organic ingredients and see the difference with these meal and juice recipes.

Almost 20% of all cancer deaths in the world, including males and females, are from breast cancer and is the most common invasive cancer in women. These rates are higher in developed nations mostly because of different lifestyle and eating habits.

In such conditions, it is imperative to have a nutrition plan, and incorporate healthy ingredients together with proper cooking techniques has been increasingly recognized as the most efficient and effective way for women as well as men to achieve optimum health results and to strengthen their immune systems.

I wanted to share with you a wonderful collection of powerful nutrition boosting recipes that will have a huge impact on different aspects of your body and health. These recipes are based on healthy fats, lean proteins, unprocessed carbs, vitamins, minerals, and other important nutrients. Each recipe is carefully designed to be delicious, easy to prepare, and healthy. Take the next step to making a lifestyle change and allowing your body to heal itself.

107 POWERFUL BREAST CANCER MEAL AND JUICE RECIPES: FIGHT BREAST CANCER BY USING NATURAL VITAMIN-RICH FOODS

FOODS

1.   Classic Tomato Soup

Ingredients:

2 lbs of tomatoes, diced

1 cup of skim milk

4 cups of chicken broth

3 garlic cloves, finely chopped

2 tbsp of fresh basil, finely chopped

1 tsp of dried oregano, ground

1 tsp of salt

¼ tsp of black pepper, ground

1 tbsp of olive oil

Preparation:

Preheat the oil in a heavy-bottomed over a medium-high temperature. Add onions and garlic and stir-fry for about 3-4 minutes, or until translucent.

Stir in the basil and oregano and simmer for 1 minute. Reduce the heat to low and add tomatoes. Pour the chicken broth and bring it to a boil. Sprinkle with salt and pepper and cook for about 13-15 minutes. Remove from the heat and set aside to cool for a while.

Transfer all to a food processor in a few batches and blend until smooth and creamy. Return to the pot and stir in the milk. Reheat and serve warm.

You can add some chili pepper if you like, but it's optional.

Garnish with fresh basil or parsley.

Nutrition information per serving: Kcal: 137, Protein: 9.1g, Carbs: 13.8g, Fats: 5.4g

2.   Al Cartoccio

Ingredients:

1 lb of chicken breasts, skinless, boneless, cut into bite-sized pieces

¼ cup of Shiitake mushrooms, chopped

¼ cup of oyster mushrooms, dried

1 cup of pumpkin, chopped

1 small celery stalk, chopped

2 garlic cloves, finely chopped

½ tsp of ginger, ground

½ tsp of salt

¼ tsp of marjoram, finely chopped

¼ cup of white wine

2 tbsp of olive oil

Preparation:

Preheat the oven to 420°F.

Peel the pumpkin and cut one large wedge. Cut into bite-sized pieces and remove the seeds. Reserve the rest in a refrigerator.

Soak the oyster mushrooms in water for 5 minutes. Drain well and set aside.

Wash the chicken breasts under cold running water and cut into bite-sized pieces.

Now, combine all ingredients in a large bowl. Stir until well incorporated.

Use a large piece of parchment paper and fold in half all the edges so that you make something lake a bag. Hold all edges in hand and place all ingredients in it. The best way is to ask someone to help you. Using a kitchen twine, gently tide up the edges so the ingredients don't come out.

Place the bag on a large baking sheet and place it in the oven. Bake for about 25-30 minutes. Remove from the heat and set aside to cool for a while.

Open the bag and transfer to a serving plate. Enjoy!

Nutrition information per serving: Kcal: 353, Protein: 36.7g, Carbs: 13.1g, Fats: 15.6g

3.   Kiwi Pear Smoothie

Ingredients:

2 large kiwis, peeled

1 large pear, chopped

1 cup of blueberries, chopped

1 cup of Greek yogurt

1 tbsp of honey, raw

1 tbsp of chia seeds

Preparation:

Peel the kiwis and cut lengthwise in half. Set aside.

Wash the pear and cut in half. Remove the core and cut into bite-sized pieces. Set aside.

Using a colander, rinse the blueberries under cold running water. Drain and set aside.

Now, combine kiwis, pear, blueberries, yogurt, honey, and chia seeds in a food processor. Blend until creamy and smooth. Transfer to serving glasses and top with chia seeds.

Refrigerate for 15 minutes before serving.

Enjoy!

Nutrition information per serving: Kcal: 314, Protein: 14.9g, Carbs: 50.2g, Fats: 7.6g

4.   Chicken Zucchini Porridge

Ingredients:

1 lb of chicken fillets, cut into bite-sized pieces

1 small zucchini, peeled and chopped

1 cup of fresh broccoli, chopped

2 tbsp of olive oil

½ tsp of salt

Preparation:

Wash the broccoli and cut into bite-sized pieces. Set aside.

Peel the zucchini and cut into small chunks. Set aside.

Wash the meat under cold running water. Pat dry and cut into bite-sized pieces. Place the meat chops in a deep pot. Add enough water to cover all and bring it to a boil. Cook for 10 minutes and then reduce the heat. Add broccoli and zucchini and stir well.

Cook for about 20-25 minutes. Remove from heat and transfer to a food processor and blend until smooth. Return to the pot and stir in the pot. Sprinkle with salt and serve warm.

Nutrition information per serving: Kcal: 384, Protein: 45.1g, Carbs: 3.3g, Fats: 20.7g

5.   Spicy Tuna with Coriander

Ingredients:

4 medium-sized tuna steaks, about 2lbs

¼ cup of fresh coriander, chopped

3 garlic cloves, minced

2 tbsp of lemon juice, freshly squeezed

½ cup olive oil

½ tsp of smoked paprika, ground

½ tsp of cumin, ground

½ tsp of chili powder

1 tsp of salt

¼ tsp of black pepper, freshly ground

Preparation:

Combine coriander, garlic, paprika, cumin, chili, and lemon juice in a food processor. Blend to combine and gradually add the olive oil. Mix the ingredients until a smooth and creamy.

Transfer the mixture into a bowl, add the fish and gently

toss to coat the fish evenly with sauce. Chill for at least 2 hours to allow the flavors to penetrate into the fish.

Preheat the grill to a medium-high heat.

Remove the fish from the chiller. Lightly brush the grid with oil, place the fish and grill for about 3-4 minutes on each side.

Remove the fish from the grill, transfer to a serving plate and serve with lemon wedges or steamed vegetables. However, it's optional.

Enjoy!

Nutrition information per serving: Kcal: 520, Protein: 60.5g, Carbs: 1.5g, Fats: 29.1g

6.   Spinach on Malaysian Way

Ingredients:

1 lb of fresh spinach, finely chopped

½ cup of spring onions, chopped

1 tsp of cayenne pepper, ground

¼ tsp of chili pepper, ground

2 tbsp of peanuts, minced

2 garlic cloves, crushed

1 small onion, chopped

2 tbsp of lemon juice, freshly squeezed

½ tsp of salt

2 tbsp of olive oil

Preparation:

Wash the spinach thoroughly under cold running water. Drain and place in a pot of boiling water. Cook for 1 minute and remove from the heat. Drain well again and finely chop it.

In a large saucepan, heat up the oil over a medium-high temperature. Add onions and spring onions. Sprinkle with cayenne, chili, and salt. Stir-fry for 3 minutes and then add peanuts. Cook for 2 more minutes and then add spinach.

Sprinkle with lemon juice and cook for 1 more minute. Remove from the heat and give it a good stir.

Serve immediately.

Nutrition information per serving: Kcal: 257, Protein: 10.1g, Carbs: 16.7g, Fats: 19.8g

7. Blueberry Sorbet

Ingredients:

2 cups of fresh blueberries

1 tsp of vanilla extract

2 tsp of white rum

1 large lemon, peeled and juiced

1 cup of water

Preparation:

Place the blueberries in a colander and rinse under cold running water. Drain and place in a deep pot.

Add vanilla extract and rum. Stir until well incorporated and bring it to a boil. Remove from the heat and drizzle with lemon juice. Set aside and allow it to cool completely.

Pour in a glass bowl and refrigerate for at least 3 hours. Stir few times while freezing. Place the glasses in the refrigerator 15 minutes before serving. Top with some fresh blueberries and enjoy!

Nutrition information per serving: Kcal: 108, Protein: 1.4g, Carbs: 24g, Fats: 0.6g

8.   Rice with Carrots and Zucchini

Ingredients:

1 cup of brown rice

1 medium-sized carrot, sliced

1 medium-sized zucchini, sliced

1 small tomato, roughly chopped

½ small eggplant, sliced

1 small red pepper, sliced

3 tbsp of extra-virgin olive oil

½ tsp of salt

1 tsp of dry marjoram

Preparation:

Place the rice in a deep pot. Add 2 cups of water and bring it to a boil. Reduce the heat and cook until the water evaporates. Stir occasionally.

Heat up one tablespoon of olive oil over a medium-high heat. Add sliced carrot and stir-fry for 3-4 minutes, stirring constantly. Combine with rice.

Stir in the remaining olive oil, zucchini, tomato, eggpla
red pepper, salt, and marjoram. Add one cup of water a
continue to cook for another 10 minutes.

Nutrition information per serving: Kcal: 220, Protein: 6g,
Carbs: 51g, Fats: 7.8g

9.   Chicken Breasts with Garlic

Ingredients:

2 chicken breast halves, skinless and boneless

½ cup of extra virgin olive oil

3 garlic cloves, crushed

½ cup of fresh parsley leaves

1 tbsp of fresh lime juice

¼ tsp of salt

Preparation:

Combine the olive oil with crushed garlic cloves, finely chopped parsley, fresh lime juice, and salt. Wash and pat dry the meat and cut into 1 inch-thick slices.

With a kitchen brush, spread the olive oil mixture over the meat. Let it stand for about 15 minutes.

Preheat the grill pan over a medium temperature. Add some marinade in the grill pan - about 2 tablespoons. Place the meat in it and grill on both sides, until lightly charred.

Remove from the pan and serve with some fresh vegetables of your choice.

Nutrition information per serving: Kcal: 485, Protein: 28.7g, Carbs: 2.9g, Fats: 40.9g

10.   Lentils with Tomato Mushroom Sauce

Ingredients:

1 lb of green lentils, soaked overnight

1 cup of button mushrooms, chopped

1 cup of tomatoes, diced

1 tbsp of fresh basil, finely chopped

2 tbsp of olive oil

2 tbsp of white wine

1 tsp of cayenne pepper, ground

½ tsp of salt

¼ tsp of dried oregano

Preparation:

Wash the mushrooms and cut the stems. Cut into bite-sized pieces and set aside.

Wash the tomatoes and place them in a blender. Add oregano and pulse until blended. Set aside.

Soak the lentils overnight. Drain and rinse well. Place it in a deep pot and add 3 cups of water. Bring it to a boil and cook for 20 minutes, or until soften. Reduce the heat to low.

Meanwhile, preheat the oil in a large saucepan over a medium-high temperature. Add mushrooms and cook for 3 minutes and then add tomatoes. Sprinkle with salt and stir well. Cook for 3 minutes and remove from the heat. Pour this mixture into the lentil pot. Sprinkle with cayenne pepper and stir well. Add more water to adjust the thickness, if needed. Bring it to a boil and cook for 10 minutes more. Remove from the heat and serve with polenta or pasta.

Sprinkle some parmesan cheese for some extra taste, but it's optional.

Nutrition information per serving: Kcal: 480, Protein: 30.3g, Carbs: 24g, Fats: 0.6g

11.　Lemon Broccoli

Ingredients:

1 lb of fresh broccoli, chopped

¼ cup of fresh parsley, finely chopped

1 tsp of dry thyme, ground

1 tbsp of lemon juice, freshly squeezed

¼ tsp of chili pepper, ground

3 tbsp of olive oil

1 tbsp of cashew cream

Preparation:

Place the broccoli in a deep pot and pour enough water to cover. Bring it to a boil and cook until tender. Remove from the heat and drain.

Transfer to a food processor. Add fresh parsley, thyme, and about ½ cup of water. Blend until nicely smooth and creamy. Return to a pot and add some more water. Bring it to a boil and cook for several minutes, over a minimum temperature.

Stir in some olive oil and cashew cream, sprinkle with

ground chili pepper and add fresh lemon juice. Serve warm.

Nutrition information per serving: Kcal: 181, Protein: 4.5g, Carbs: 11.1g, Fats: 14.9g

12.   Lentil Red Pepper Salad

Ingredients:

1 cup of lentils, soaked and pre-cooked

1 medium-sized red bell pepper, chopped

½ cup of sweet corn

A handful of purple cabbage, shredded

A handful of lettuce, shredded

½ tsp of salt

¼ tsp of black pepper, freshly ground

2 tbsp of olive oil

1 tbsp of sesame seeds

Preparation:

Wash and prepare the vegetables.

Soak the lentil overnight. Drain and rinse well. Drain again and place the lentils in a deep pot. Use 3 cups of water for 1 cup of dry lentils.

Bring it to a boil and then reduce the heat to medium. Cover with a lid and cook for about 15-20 minutes. Remove from the heat and drain. Transfer to a bowl.

Now add bell peppers, corn, cabbage, and lettuce. Sprinkle with salt, pepper, olive oil, and sprinkle with sesame seeds. Toss well to combine.

Nutrition information per serving: Kcal: 272, Protein: 13.9g, Carbs: 36.2g, Fats: 9g

13.   Turkey Thighs in Garlic Sauce

Ingredients:

1 lb of turkey thighs

1 large red onion, chopped

4 garlic cloves, crushed

½ cup of celery, chopped

½ cup of red wine

1 cup of chicken broth

1 tbsp of olive oil

½ tsp of salt

½ tsp of black pepper, ground

Preparation:

Wash the turkey thighs and pat dry with a kitchen paper. Cut each thigh in half and set aside.

Preheat the oil in a large saucepan over a medium-high temperature. Add thighs and cook for about 4-5 minutes on each side. Remove the thighs from the saucepan and set aside.

In the same saucepan, add onions, celery, and garlic. Stir-fry for 5 minutes, or until onions translucent. Now, return the thighs to the saucepan and pour the broth and wine. Bring it to a boil and then reduce the heat to low. Cook for 30 minutes. Add hot water if needed while cooking. Remove from the heat and serve warm.

Nutrition information per serving: Kcal: 263, Protein: 12.9g, Carbs: 12.1g, Fats: 13.9g

14.   Egg-Carrot Spaghetti

Ingredients:

1 lb of spaghetti pasta

1 large carrot, grated

1 large egg, beaten

1 tbsp of olive oil

½ tsp of dried oregano, ground

½ tsp of salt

¼ tsp of black pepper, ground

Preparation:

Cook the spaghetti using package instructions. Drain well and set aside.

Peel the carrot and grate it. Set aside.

Whisk the eggs with salt, oregano, and pepper. Set aside.

Now, preheat the oil in a large skillet over a medium-high temperature. Add grated carrot and sprinkle with salt and pepper. Cook for 2 minutes, stirring occasionally. Add pasta and pour the egg mixture. Stir and cook for about 3-4 minutes, or until the eggs are set.

Remove from the heat and serve with some fresh salad or sprinkle with grated Parmesan cheese.

Enjoy!

Nutrition information per serving: Kcal: 348, Protein: 11.2g, Carbs: 49.4g, Fats: 11.6g

15.   Kale with Chicken and Potatoes

Ingredients:

1 lb of fresh kale, chopped

1 lb of chicken fillets, cut into bite-sized pieces

2 garlic cloves, crushed

2 medium-sized potatoes, chopped

1 small carrot, chopped

2 tbsp of sour cream

1 tbsp of all-purpose flour

1 tsp of cayenne pepper

3 tbsp of olive oil

1 tsp of salt

½ tsp of black pepper, ground

Preparation:

Wash the fillets and pat dry with a kitchen paper. Cut into bite-sized pieces and set aside.

Peel the potatoes and cut into small chunks. Place in a pot of boiling water and cook for 10 minutes, or until fork tender. Remove from the heat and drain well. Set aside.

Wash the kale thoroughly under cold running water. Drain and chop into small pieces. place it in a deep pot and add water enough to cover. Bring it to a boil and cook for about 2-3 minutes. Remove from the heat and drain well.

Preheat the oil in a large skillet over a medium-high temperature. Add onions and stir-fry until translucent. Add chopped fillets and cook for 5 minutes, stirring occasionally. Now, add ½ cup of water and then add kale and potato. Sprinkle with salt and pepper and cook for another 5 minutes. Reduce the heat to low and stir in the cayenne and flour. Cook for 2 more minutes.

Remove from the heat and serve warm.

Nutrition information per serving: Kcal: 464, Protein: 38.7g, Carbs: 32.5g, Fats: 20.4g

16.   Trout in Sour Cream Sauce

Ingredients:

1 lb of trout fillets

1 tbsp of olive oil

¼ tsp of black pepper, ground

1 large lemon, freshly juiced

½ cup of sour cream

1 medium-sized onion, chopped

1 small zucchini, chopped

1 tsp of fresh rosemary, finely chopped

Preparation:

Wash the fillets under cold water and pat dry with a kitchen paper. Set aside.

Preheat the oil in a large frying pan and add fillets. Sprinkle with salt, pepper, and rosemary. Fry for about 3-4 minutes on each side, or until golden brown. Remove from the heat and transfer to a plate. Reserve the pan.

Add lemon juice and sour cream to the pan. Simmer until the mixture thickens. Remove from the pan and transfer to a small bowl. Set aside.

Now, add onions and zucchini to the pan. Add 1 cup of water and increase the heat to high. Bring it to a boil and then cover with a lid. Cook for about 10-12 minutes, or until tender. Remove from the heat and sprinkle with some salt and pepper if you like.

Serve the fillets with vegetables and pour over the sauce.

Nutrition information per serving: Kcal: 438, Protein: 42.6g, Carbs: 8.6g, Fats: 25.8g

17.　Strawberry Mango Smoothie

Ingredients:

1 cup of fresh strawberries, chopped

1 medium-sized ripe mango, chopped

1 large banana, chopped

½ cup of skim milk

½ cup of Greek yogurt

2 tbsp of orange juice, freshly juiced

Preparation:

Wash the strawberries under cold running water. Drain and chop into bite-sized pieces. Set aside.

Peel the mango and cut into chunks. Set aside.

Peel the banana and cut into thin slices. Set aside.

Now, combine strawberries, mango, banana, milk, yogurt, and orange juice in a blender. Process until smooth and creamy. Transfer to serving glasses and add few ice cubes before serving.

Enjoy!

Nutrition information per serving: Kcal: 251, Protein: 9.8g, Carbs: 52.7g, Fats: 2.1g

18.   Green Bean Salad with Lime

Ingredients:

3 oz of green beans, cooked

3 cherry tomatoes, halved

1 small red bell pepper, chopped

1 small red onion, peeled and sliced

¼ cup of fresh lime juice

3 tbsp of olive oil

1 tsp of honey

½ small shallot, minced

1 garlic clove, crushed

¼ tsp of salt

Preparation:

Combine the lime juice with honey. Mix well with a fork. Gradually, add the olive oil, whisking constantly. Now add the minced shallot, crushed garlic clove, and salt. Set aside to allow flavors to meld.

Meanwhile, wash the green beans and place in a deep pot.

Add 3 cups of water and bring it to a boil. Cook for 15 minutes and remove from the heat. Drain well and sprinkle with some salt. Set aside.

Wash the tomatoes and cut into bite-sized pieces and set aside.

Wash the bell pepper and cut lengthwise in half. Remove the seeds and chop into small pieces. Set aside.

Peel the onion and chop into small pieces. Set aside.

Now, combine green beans, tomatoes, bell pepper, and onions. Stir once and then drizzle with the previously prepared dressing. Toss to combine and serve immediately.

Nutrition information per serving: Kcal: 275, Protein: 3.6g, Carbs: 22.2g, Fats: 21.6g

19.   Turkey with Pomegranate Sauce

Ingredients:

1 lb of turkey breasts, skinless and boneless

2 small pomegranates, whole

4 tbsp of olive oil

1 tsp of dried thyme, ground

1 tsp of salt

½ tsp of black pepper, freshly ground

Preparation:

Wash the meat under cold running water and pat dry with a kitchen paper. Gently rub with salt and pepper and set aside.

Place the pomegranate fruit between your palms and press hard. Make a small hole in the middle of the fruit and squeeze the juice to a cup. Set aside.

Using a sharp paring knife, cut the top of the remaining pomegranate. Slice down to each of the white membranes inside of the fruit. Pop the seeds into a cup or a small bowl and set aside.

Preheat the oil in a large skillet over a medium-high temperature. Add meat and cook for about 4-5 minutes on each side and then reduce the heat to low.

Drizzle the meat with freshly squeezed pomegranate juice and cook for about 1-2 minutes, or until it thickens. Sprinkle with thyme and remove from the heat. Stir in the pomegranate seeds and serve with mashed potatoes or rice.

Enjoy!

Nutrition information per serving: Kcal: 386, Protein: 26.6g, Carbs: 24.1g, Fats: 21.2g

20.   Grilled Veal with Veggies

Ingredients:

1 lb of veal steak, cut into 1-inch thick pieces

1 medium-sized red bell pepper, chopped

1 medium-sized yellow bell pepper, chopped

1 small onion, peeled and sliced

3 tbsp of olive oil

½ tsp of salt

½ tsp of black pepper, ground

Preparation:

Wash the bell peppers and cut lengthwise in half. Remove the seeds and chop into thin strips. Set aside.

Wash and pat dry the steak with a kitchen paper. Heat up the olive oil over a medium temperature and fry the meat for about 10-15 minutes (about 5-7 minutes on each side). Remove from the heat and set aside.

Place prepared vegetables in the same frying skillet and stir-fry for about 13-15 minutes. Stir occasionally. Remove from the heat and serve with meat.

Serve immediately.

Nutrition information per serving: Kcal: 309, Protein: 35.4g, Carbs: 7.1g, Fats: 17.1g

21.   Avocado Garlic Aioli

Ingredients:

2 medium-sized avocados, chopped

3 garlic cloves, peeled

2 large eggs, beaten

2 tbsp of sour cream

1 tbsp of olive oil

1 tbsp of lemon juice, freshly squeezed

½ tsp of salt

½ tsp of black pepper, ground

Preparation:

Peel the avocado and cut lengthwise in half. Remove the pits and cut into small chunks. Set aside.

Peel the garlic and roughly chop it.

Now, combine avocado, garlic, eggs, sour cream, olive oil, lemon juice, salt, and pepper in a blender. Process until well combined and creamy. Transfer to a plastic container and refrigerate for 20 minutes before serving.

Serve aioli with cooked eggs, roasted meat, or simply spread it on a bread slice. Enjoy!

Nutrition information per serving: Kcal: 385, Protein: 7.3g, Carbs: 13.5g, Fats: 35.9g

22.   Blueberry Mousse

Ingredients:

1 cup of blueberries

1 cup of strawberries, chopped

½ cup of almond milk

2 cups of coconut milk

1 oz of Greek yogurt

2 egg whites

¼ cup of almonds, roughly chopped

1 tbsp of vanilla extract

½ tsp of cinnamon, ground

Preparation:

Wash the blueberries in a colander. Slightly drain and set aside.

Wash the strawberries and cut into bite-sized pieces. Set aside.

Beat the egg whites, yogurt, and milk with a fork. It will take about 5 minutes to get a nice, smooth mousse. Pour this mousse in a blender, add blueberries, strawberries, water and mix for 20 seconds.

Add some cinnamon and vanilla extract for some extra taste. Top with roughly chopped almonds and garnish with some fresh blueberries.

Enjoy!

Nutrition information per serving: Kcal: 407, Protein: 11.6g, Carbs: 19g, Fats: 33.5g

23.   Grilled Zucchini

Ingredients:

6 oz zucchini, sliced

¼ cup of lemon juice, freshly squeezed

1 tbsp of olive oil

¼ tsp of sea salt

1 tsp dry rosemary, finely chopped

¼ tsp of black pepper, freshly ground

Preparation:

Whisk together lemon juice, sea salt, rosemary, and black pepper.

Wash and peel the zucchini. Cut into 1-inch thick slices. Brush each slice with a previously prepared mixture.

Preheat the oil in a large grill pan over a medium-high temperature. Add zucchini and grill on both sides for 4-5 minutes, or until lightly charred.

Serve as a side dish or a main meal with some sour cream.

Enjoy!

Nutrition information per serving: Kcal: 168, Protein: 2.7g, Carbs: 8.1g, Fats: 15g

24. Rigatoni with Basil Pesto

Ingredients:

1 lb of rigatoni pasta

8 oz of fresh basil, torn

3 garlic cloves, crushed

2 tbsp of pine nuts

4 tbsp of olive oil

4 tbsp of Parmesan cheese, grated

1 tsp of sea salt

Preparation:

Wash the basil thoroughly under cold running water.Drain and transfer to a large kitchen cloth or a piece of paper. Pat dry and roughly chop it.

Crush the garlic in the mortar and sprinkle with some salt. Gradually add basil and crush it. When crushing basil, make circle moves to get an essential aroma out of it.

Add pine nuts to the mortar and gently crush it and combine with the basil pesto. Now, transfer all to a large bowl and add cheese and olive oil. Stir until well combined. Set aside.

Cook the pasta using package instructions. Drain well and transfer to a serving bowl. Add basil pesto and stir well.

Garnish with some fresh basil leaves and sprinkle with salt to taste.

Nutrition information per serving: Kcal: 514, Protein: 17.6g, Carbs: 65.1g, Fats: 21.4g

25.   Mango Peach Smoothie

Ingredients:

1 medium-sized mango, chopped

1 large peach, pitted and chopped

1 large carrot, sliced

1 tbsp of honey, raw

2 oz of water

Preparation:

Wash the mango and cut into bite-sized pieces. Set aside.

Wash the peach and cut in half. Remove the pit and cut into small pieces. Set aside.

Wash and peel the carrot. Cut into thin slices and set aside.

Now, combine mango, peach, carrot, honey, and water in a food processor. Blend until nicely smooth and transfer to serving glasses.

Add some ice, or refrigerate for about 15-20 minutes before serving.

Enjoy!

Nutrition information per serving: Kcal: 353, Protein: 4.9g, Carbs: 88.4g, Fats: 1.7g

26.   Banana-Berry Porridge

Ingredients:

1 cup of quinoa

½ cup of almond milk

3 cups of water

1 small banana, peeled and sliced

2 tbsp of blueberries

1 tbsp of honey

2 tsp of chia seeds, soaked

2 tbsp of almonds, roughly chopped

Preparation:

Combine water and almond milk in a medium saucepan and heat up over medium-high temperature. Bring it to a boil and add quinoa. Reduce the heat to low and cook for about 15-20 minutes.

Meanwhile, mash the banana with a fork and roughly chop the almonds. Set aside.

Transfer the cooked quinoa to a bowl. Stir in the mashed banana, blueberries, honey, and chia seeds.

Top with sliced banana and chopped almonds.

Nutrition information per serving: Kcal: 362, Protein: 10.8g, Carbs: 45.6, Fats: 16.1g

27. Veal Carrot Stew

Ingredients:

2 lbs of veal steak, cut into bite-sized pieces

1 large carrot, sliced

2 medium-sized tomatoes, diced

1 tbsp of tomato paste

4 cups of beef broth

2 tbsp of olive oil

1 tsp of dried thyme, ground

1 tsp of salt

½ tsp of black pepper, ground

Preparation:

Wash the meat thoroughly under cold running water. Pat dry with a kitchen paper and cut into bite-sized pieces. Place in a deep bowl and sprinkle with salt and pepper. Mix with hands until well incorporated. Set aside.

Preheat the oil in a large skillet over a medium-high temperature. Add meat chops and cook for 10 minutes, or until golden brown. Stir occasionally.

Peel the carrot and cut into thin slices. Add it to the skillet with meat and stir well.

Add the broth and bring it to a boil. Reduce the heat to low and simmer for 10 more minutes. Add diced tomatoes and tomato paste. Stir well and cook for 5 more minutes. Sprinkle with more salt and pepper if needed and remove from the heat.

Serve with cooked rice. However, this is optional.

Nutrition information per serving: Kcal: 415, Protein: 52.4g, Carbs: 4.9g, Fats: 19.4g

28.   Salmon with Honey and Coriander

Ingredients:

1 lb of salmon fillets

1 tbsp of coriander seeds

4 tbsp of honey, raw

½ cup of fish sauce

2 tbsp of lemon juice, freshly squeezed

2 tbsp of olive oil

½ tsp of sea salt

½ tsp of black pepper, ground

Preparation:

Wash the fillets under cold running water and pat dry with a kitchen paper. Set aside.

Place coriander seeds in a dry frying pan. Fry for 2-3 minutes on a medium-high temperature. Remove from the heat and let it cool completely. Using a mortar and pestle, crush into nice powder. Set aside.

In a medium bowl, combine honey, fish sauce, lemon juice, and 1 tablespoon of olive oil. Add coriander powder and stir until all well combined. Now, spread this cream over the fish fillets.

Preheat the remaining oil in a large skillet over a medium-high temperature. Add prepared fillets and cook for 2 minutes. Reduce the heat and cook for 1 more minute. Turn the fillets and cook for 3 minutes more.

Serve the salmon with steamed vegetables like broccoli, asparagus, or baked sweet potatoes. However, it's optional.

Enjoy!

Nutrition information per serving: Kcal: 385, Protein: 32g, Carbs: 25.3g, Fats: 18.8g

29.   Blueberry Buckwheat Pancakes

Ingredients:

4 tbsp buckwheat flour

4 large eggs

4 tbsp flax seeds, minced

1 cup of almond milk

¼ tsp of salt

1 cup of Greek yogurt

1 cup of fresh blueberries

1 tbsp of canola oil

Preparation:

Combine the ingredients in a bowl. Beat well with an electric mixer, on high.

Heat up the oil in a medium skillet over a medium-high temperature. Pour some of the mixture in the skillet and fry the pancakes for about 2-3 minutes, on each side.

Using a colander, wash the blueberries under cold running water. Drain and set aside.

In a medium bowl, combine blueberries and yogurt. Stir until combined and spread over each pancake.

Garnish with some fresh blueberries and serve immediately.

Nutrition information per serving: Kcal: 161, Protein: 16.5g, Carbs: 10g, Fats: 5g

30.   Rye Carrot Muffins

Ingredients:

1 cup of rye flour

1 tbsp of corn flour

3 large carrots, sliced

1 medium-sized red onion, chopped

1 oz capers, drained

1 tbsp of sesame seeds

1 tbsp of flaxseeds

1 tsp of baking soda

½ tsp of curry, ground

½ tsp of salt

2 tsp of olive oil

Preparation:

Preheat the oven to 375°F.

In a large bowl, combine rye flour, corn flour, baking soda, curry, and salt. Stir until well incorporated and set aside.

Combine onion, sesame seeds, and flax seeds in a medium frying pan. Heat up over a medium-high temperature and add capers. Stir-fry for about 3-4 minutes, or until the onions translucent. Reduce the heat and stir in the carrot. Fry for 2 more minutes and remove from the heat. Add this mixture to dry ingredients and stir all well until combined.

Grease muffin molds with some olive oil. Spoon the mixture into the molds and place it in the oven.

Bake for about 10-15 minutes, or until nicely browned. Remove from the heat and allow it to cool for a while.

Enjoy!

Nutrition information per serving: Kcal: 150, Protein: 5g, Carbs: 26.2g, Fats: 4.1g

31. Vegetable Mozzarella Salad

Ingredients:

1 small zucchini, chopped

2 large red bell peppers, chopped

1 cup of eggplants, chopped

½ cup of Mozzarella

1 oz of fresh basil, finely chopped

4 tbsp of olive oil

1 tbsp of balsamic vinegar

½ tsp of garlic powder

1 tsp of Italian seasoning

½ tsp of salt

½ tsp of black pepper, freshly ground

Preparation:

Wash the zucchini and cut into thin slices. Set aside.

Wash the bell peppers and cut in half lengthwise. Remove the seeds and cut into small pieces. Set aside.

Wash the eggplant and cut into small chunks. Set aside.

Now, preheat 1 tablespoon of olive oil in a large frying pan. Add zucchini, bell peppers, and eggplant. Cook for 5 minutes, stirring occasionally.

Meanwhile, combine basil, garlic, vinegar, salt, pepper, and the remaining oil in a medium bowl. Stir until well incorporated. Set aside.

Transfer cooked vegetables to a large bowl. Top with crumbled Mozzarella and drizzle with previously prepared dressing.

Garnish with fresh basil leaves and enjoy.

Nutrition information per serving: Kcal: 333, Protein: 5.1g, Carbs: 15.2g, Fats: 30.6g

32.   Southern Style Chicken

Ingredients:

1 lb of chicken breasts, skinless and boneless

1 tsp of Worcestershire sauce

1 tsp of molasses

2 large tomatoes, diced

1 tbsp of tomato paste

2 garlic cloves, minced

½ tsp of black pepper, freshly ground

½ tsp of cayenne pepper, ground

½ tsp of salt

Preparation:

Preheat the oven to 350°F.

Wash the chicken under cold running water and pat dry with a kitchen paper. Cut into thin slices and set aside.

In a large saucepan, combine Worcestershire sauce, molasses, tomatoes, tomato paste, and cayenne pepper. Simmer for 10 minutes over a medium-high temperature.

Remove from the heat and transfer to a large bowl. Add chicken and refrigerate to marinate for at least 1 hour.

Line some aluminum foil over a medium baking sheet and add chicken breasts. Pour the sauce and spread evenly. Cover all with another piece of aluminum foil and place it in the oven.

Bake for about 35-40 minutes, or until nicely golden brown. Remove from the heat and transfer to serving plate. Serve with rice or steamed vegetables.

Enjoy!

Nutrition information per serving: Kcal: 326, Protein: 45.3g, Carbs: 8.8g, Fats: 11.5g

33.   Spinach and Goat's Cheese Omelet

Ingredients:

4 large eggs, beaten

1 oz fresh goat's cheese, crumbled

1 medium-sized onion, peeled and chopped

1 cup of fresh spinach, finely chopped

2 tbsp of extra-virgin olive oil

½ tsp of salt

Preparation:

Wash the spinach thoroughly under cold running water. Chop into small pieces and place in a pot of boiling water. Cook for 2 minutes and remove from the heat.

Preheat the olive oil in a large frying pan over a medium-high temperature. Add onions and stir-fry for about 3-4 minutes, or until translucent.

Crack the eggs in a large bowl. Sprinkle with some salt and mix well with a fork. Whisk in the spinach and cheese.

Pour the egg mixture and spread evenly in a pan. Cook for about 4-5 minutes, or until the eggs are set.

Nutrition information per serving: Kcal: 340, Protein: 16.7g, Carbs: 6.8g, Fats: 28.3g

34.   Mixed Berries Smoothie

Ingredients:

½ cup of blueberries

½ cup of blackberries

½ cup of skim milk

¼ cup of lemon juice, freshly squeezed

1 tbsp of honey, raw

Preparation:

Combine blueberries and blackberries in a large colander. Rinse under cold running water and slightly drain. Transfer to a food processor and add milk, fresh lemon juice, and honey.

Blend until nicely smooth and creamy.

Transfer to serving glasses and garnish with some fresh berries and lemon slices. Add some ice or refrigerate for 10 minutes before serving.

Enjoy!

Nutrition information per serving: Kcal: 196, Protein: 6.1g, Carbs: 42g, Fats: 1.1g

35.   Veal with Tuna Spread

Ingredients:

1 lb of veal steak, cut into bite-sized pieces

1 medium-sized onion, chopped

1 medium-sized celery stalk, chopped

½ tsp of salt

1 cup of tuna, minced

1 tbsp of capers, drained

1 large lemon, freshly juiced

1 cup of chicken broth

Preparation:

Wash the meat under cold running water and pat dry with a kitchen paper. Cut into bite-sized pieces.

Place the meat in a deep pot. Add water enough to cover and bring it to a boil. Add onions, celery, and salt. Cook for about 40-45 minutes and then remove from the heat. Remove the meat from the pot and place it on a plate. Refrigerate overnight.

Combine tuna and capers in a medium bowl. Add lemon

juice and about 2-3 tablespoons of the liquid from the pot. Give it a good stir and chill out for a couple of minutes.

Now, cut the meat into very thin slices and transfer to a serving plate. Top with tuna spread. Garnish with olives or fresh parsley and enjoy.

Nutrition information per serving: Kcal: 411, Protein: 57.9g, Carbs: 6.1g, Fats: 15.9g

36.   Sweet Apple Cider

Ingredients:

2 lbs of Fuji apples, wedged

½ cup of honey, raw

¼ tsp of cinnamon, ground

4 cups of water

Preparation:

Wash the apples and cut lengthwise in half. Remove the seeds and cut into wedges. Place the apples in a deep pot. Add water enough to cover all and stir in the honey and cinnamon.

Bring it to a boil and then reduce the heat to low. Cook for 3 hours, or until soften and light browned. Remove from the heat and let it cool for a while.

Using a small colander, squeeze the juice into a bowl. Taste and add more honey or cinnamon if you like. This is optional.

Refrigerate for 30 minutes before serving. You can keep the juice up to 2 days in the refrigerator.

Nutrition information per serving: Kcal: 187, Protein: 0.4g, Carbs: 50.4g, Fats: 0.2g

37.   Apricot Oatmeal with Seeds

Ingredients:

1 cup of rolled oats

1 cup of skim milk

1 medium-sized apricot, chopped

1 tbsp of chia seeds

1 tbsp of flaxseeds, minced

2 tbsp of honey

1 tsp of cocoa, raw

¼ tsp of cinnamon, ground

Preparation:

In a medium pot, combine rolled oats, milk, cocoa, and cinnamon. Stir well and bring it to a boil. Remove from the heat and fluff with a fork. Set aside to soak for 10 minutes.

Meanwhile, wash the apricot and cut lengthwise in half. Remove the pit and cut into bite-sized pieces. Set aside.

Now, stir in the honey, apricots, and flaxseeds in oatmeal. Top with chia and any fresh fruit of your choice.

Serve cold.

Nutrition information per serving: Kcal: 371, Protein: 13.6g, Carbs: 59.9, Fats: 8.8g

38.   Mascarpone Coffee Smoothie

Ingredients:

½ cup of Mascarpone cheese

½ cup of skim milk

1 tsp of vanilla extract

1 tbsp of black coffee powder

1 tbsp of cocoa, raw

2 tbsp of chocolate chips

Preparation:

Combine coffee powder with 4 tbsp of water in a small pot. Bring it to a boil and set aside.

In a blender, combine cheese, milk, vanilla extract. Blend well and transfer to small bowl. Clean the blender and place coffee, cocoa and chocolate chips. Blend until smooth and creamy.

Now, first fill the serving glass with black mixture and top with white cheese mixture.

If you like, you can stir it and sprinkle with some cocoa. Refrigerate for 30 minutes before serving.

Enjoy!

Nutrition information per serving: Kcal: 397, Protein: 20.6g, Carbs: 25.7, Fats: 23g

39. Pineapple Chicken in Sweet-Sour Sauce

Ingredients:

2 lbs of chicken fillets

1 tbsp of coconut oil

1 tsp of sesame seeds

2 tsp of flaxseeds

2 tbsp of honey

2 tbsp of tartar sauce

1 large red bell pepper, chopped

1 medium-sized onion, chopped

½ cup of pineapple, chunked

1 oz of Feta cheese

½ tsp of curry powder

½ tsp of ginger, ground

¼ tsp of chili pepper, ground

Preparation:

Wash the fillets under cold running water and pat dry with

a kitchen paper. Cut into bite-sized pieces and place in a large bowl. Add honey and tartar sauce. Stir all well and wrap the top of the bowl with a plastic foil. Refrigerate for about 30 minutes.

Wash the bell pepper and cut lengthwise in half. Remove the seeds and chop into bite-sized pieces. Peel the onion and finely chop it.

Preheat the coconut oil in a large skillet over a medium-high temperature. Add onions, pepper, and sesame seeds. Stir-fry for about 3-4 minutes and then add meat along with juices. Sprinkle with flaxseeds and simmer for about 8-10 minutes, or until golden brown.

Now, add 2 cups of hot water and pineapple chunks. Sprinkle with curry and ginger. Reduce the heat to low and simmer for 10 minutes, or until the liquid thickens.

Remove from the heat and serve immediately. Top with Feta cheese and chili pepper.

Nutrition information per serving: Kcal: 571, Protein: 67.8g, Carbs: 18.1, Fats: 24.4g

40.   Kalamari Vegetable Salad

Ingredients:

1 lb of squids, cut into rings

1 tsp of coriander, finely chopped

½ tsp of chili pepper, ground

½ tsp of sea salt

1 tbsp of balsamic vinegar

1 lime, freshly juiced

1 cup of Romaine lettuce, chopped

1 medium-sized radish, chopped

½ cup of spring onions, chopped

½ cup of arugula, chopped

2 small tomatoes, chopped

1 tbsp of olive oil

Preparation:

Wash the squids and pat dry with a kitchen paper. Cut into rings and set aside.

Preheat the oil in a large frying pan over a medium-high temperature. Add balsamic vinegar, coriander, lime juice, and chili pepper. Add squid rings and cook for about 4-5 minutes. Add ½ cup of water and simmer for 15 minutes. Reduce the heat to low and cook until it nicely thickens. Remove from the heat and set aside.

Wash and prepare the vegetables.

Wash the lettuce and arugula thoroughly under cold running water. Roughly chop it and place in a large bowl.

Rinse the spring onions and chop into bite-sized pieces. Add it to the bowl.

Wash the radishes and trim off the green ends. Cut into bite-sized pieces and add it to the bowl.

Wash the tomatoes and cut into small pieces. Make sure to reserve the juice while cutting. Add it to the bowl.

Now, add squid rings and stir all well. Season with some extra salt, pepper, and olive oil.

Serve immediately.

Nutrition information per serving: Kcal: 311, Protein: 37.1g, Carbs: 17.2, Fats: 10.5g

41.   Cauliflower in Dill Sauce

Ingredients:

2 cups of cauliflower, chopped

1 large egg

½ cup of Greek yogurt

2 tbsp of corn flour

1 tsp of dried parsley, ground

¼ tsp of black pepper, ground

For the sauce:

1 tsp of butter

1tbsp of all-purpose flour

¼ cup of skim milk

3 tbsp of fresh dill, finely chopped

1 tsp of red wine vinegar

1 tsp of salt

Preparation:

Wash the cauliflower under cold running water. Cut into

small florets, or chop into bite-sized pieces. Set aside.

Place the cauliflower in a deep pot. Add water enough to cover and bring it to a boil. Cook for 5 minutes and then remove from the heat. Drain well and rinse again under cold water. Drain and set aside.

In a medium bowl, combine corn flour, egg, yogurt, salt, pepper, and parsley. Stir well until you get nice batter. Set aside.

Grease the baking sheet with some oil. Pour the corn flour mixture and spread evenly on the sheet. Spread the cooked cauliflower and sprinkle with some fresh parsley and Parmesan cheese for some extra taste. However, it's optional.

Place it in the oven and bake for 20 minutes, or until nicely crisp.

Meanwhile, melt the butter in a medium frying pan over a medium-high temperature. Add flour and stir-fry for 1 minute. Add vinegar, milk, and dill. Stir well and reduce the heat to low. Cook for 2 minutes and remove from the heat.

When baked, remove the sheet from the oven and pour the prepared sauce evenly.

Set aside to soak for 10 minutes and then serve.

Nutrition information per serving: Kcal: 180, Protein: 13.1g, Carbs: 20.4g, Fats: 6g

42.   Green Pepper Eggs

Ingredients:

1 large green bell pepper, cut into thick rings

4 large eggs, whole

1 tbsp of olive oil

1 tbsp chia seeds

¼ tsp of black pepper, ground

½ tsp of salt

Preparation:

Wash the bell pepper and cut the top. Remove the seeds and cut into thick pieces. Set aside.

Preheat the oil in a large frying pan over a medium-high temperature. Add sliced peppers and crack each egg into each slice. Sprinkle with salt and pepper and cook for about 3-4 minutes, or until the eggs are set. Sprinkle with chia seeds for some extra nutrients and remove from the heat.

Using a large spatula, transfer the pepper eggs to a serving plate.

Enjoy!

Nutrition information per serving: Kcal: 301, Protein: 16.4g, Carbs: 10.7g, Fats: 21.9g

43.   Salmon with Basil Cream and Gorgonzola

Ingredients:

1 lb of salmon fillets

2 cups of asparagus, chopped

1 cup of olive oil

½ cup of fresh basil, finely chopped

½ cup of Gorgonzola cheese, crumbled

¼ cup of Greek yogurt

½ cup of sour cream

1 tbsp of shallots, finely chopped

1 tbsp of yellow mustard

1 oz of walnuts, roughly chopped

½ tsp of freshly ground black pepper

Preparation:

Preheat the oven to 450 degrees.

Place some baking paper on a large baking sheet and set aside.

Wash the fillets thoroughly under cold running water and pat dry with a kitchen paper. Set aside.

Combine walnuts, basil, olive oil, and pepper in a food processor. Blend until nicely pureed. Transfer it to a large bowl and add salmon fillets. Soak for 30 minutes before preparation.

Wash the asparagus and place them in a pot of boiling water. Cook for 2 minutes and remove from the heat. Drain well and rinse under cold running water immediately. Set aside.

In a large bowl, combine cheese, sour cream, and shallots. Stir until well incorporated. Set aside.

Place the soaked salmon fillets on a large baking sheet. Spread the mustard o the top of each fillet. Now spread the basil cream on each and place it in the oven. Bake for about 8-10 minutes.

Remove from the heat and transfer to a serving plate. Add asparagus and serve with cheese sauce.

Nutrition information per serving: Kcal: 447, Protein: 32.4g, Carbs: 7.2g, Fats: 34.2g

44.   Broccoli Fussili

Ingredients:

1 lb of fusilli pasta, pre-cooked

1 lb of fresh broccoli, chopped

2 tbsp of olive oil

1 medium-sized zucchini, chopped

2 garlic cloves, minced

2 cups of water

½ cup of sour cream

½ tsp of salt

¼ tsp of black pepper, ground

Preparation:

Cook the pasta according to package instructions. Add a pinch of salt when boiled. Remove from the heat and drain well. Set aside.

Wash the broccoli under cold running water and drain well. Chop into bite-sized pieces and place in a deep pot. Add water enough to cover and bring it to a boil. Cook for about

2-3 minutes and remove from the heat. Drain well and set aside.

Preheat the oil in a large skillet over a medium-high temperature. Add garlic and stir-fry for 2 minutes and then add chopped zucchini. Now, add water and bring it to a boil. Stir in the sour cream and cook for about 5-7 minutes. Now, add pasta and broccoli. Stir until all well incorporated.

Sprinkle with Italian seasoning, salt, and pepper to taste.

Serve immediately.

Nutrition information per serving: Kcal: 571, Protein: 19.5g, Carbs: 95g, Fats: 14.8g

45.   Radish Arugula Salad

Ingredients:

1 large Romaine lettuce head, roughly chopped

2 medium-sized radishes, chopped

1 cup of arugula, chopped

1 tbsp of walnuts, roughly chopped

1 cup of cream

¼ cup of goat's cheese

1 tbsp of honey, raw

1 tbsp of balsamic vinegar

½ tsp of salt

½ tsp of black pepper, ground

Preparation:

Wash the lettuce thoroughly under cold running water. Roughly chop it into small pieces and place in a large bowl. Set aside.

Wash the radishes and trim off the green ends. Chop into small pieces and add it to the bowl.

Wash the arugula and chop into small pieces. Add it to the bowl.

In a medium saucepan, add cream, cheese, and honey. Heat up over a medium-high temperature. Stir in the balsamic vinegar, salt, and pepper. Remove from the heat and let it cool for a while.

Now, pour the sauce over the salad and stir all well. Refrigerate for 10 minutes before serving.

Nutrition information per serving: Kcal: 207, Protein: 6.5g, Carbs: 17.1g, Fats: 13.6g

46.   Cod Spread

Ingredients:

2 lbs of cod fillets

3 garlic cloves, finely chopped

1 small onion, finely chopped

3 tbsp of olive oil

1 tsp of rosemary, finely chopped

½ cup of cream cheese

1 tsp of dried basil, ground

1 tsp of salt

¼ tsp of black pepper, ground

Preparation:

Wash the fillets thoroughly under cold running water. Cut into bite-sized pieces and remove the skin. Set aside.

Preheat 1 tablespoon of oil in a large frying pan over a medium-high temperature. Add onions and stir-fry for about 3-4 minutes. Add garlic and cook for 1 minute more. Now, add fish and sprinkle with some salt. Cook for 5 minutes, or until golden brown. Remove from the heat and set aside to cool for a while.

Now, transfer the fish with all its liquid to a food processor. Add rosemary, cream cheese, basil, salt, pepper and 1 tablespoon of oil. Blend for 2 minutes and then add remaining oil. Again, blend until well incorporated and creamy.

Serve with fresh carrots or bread slices.

Enjoy!

Nutrition information per serving: Kcal: 349, Protein: 19.5g, Carbs: 36.1g, Fats: 14.7g

47.   Oven-Baked Turkey with Citrus

Ingredients:

1 lb of turkey fillets, cut into bite-sized pieces

2 large lemons, sliced

2 large oranges, sliced

1 medium-sized onion, sliced

4 garlic cloves, finely chopped

3 tbsp of olive oil

½ tsp of salt

¼ tsp of black pepper, ground

1 tsp of Italian seasoning

½ tsp of dried thyme, ground

½ tsp of Cayenne pepper, ground

1 tbsp of fresh parsley, finely chopped

Preparation:

Preheat the oven to 400 degrees.

Wash the meat under cold running water and pat dry with a kitchen paper. Cut into bite-sized pieces and set aside.

Wash 1 lemon and 1 orange and cut into thin slices, without peeling. Set aside.

Peel the remaining lemon and juice them. Set aside.

In a medium bowl, combine lemon juice, orange juice, oil, salt, pepper, and garlic. Stir until well incorporated and pour over the turkey. Set aside to marinate for about 15-20 minutes.

In a small bowl, combine Italian seasoning, thyme, and cayenne pepper. Set aside.

Transfer the meat to a large baking sheet and tuck in the lemon and orange slices. Pour the remaining marinade and spice mixture. Sprinkle all again with some salt and pepper and place it in the oven.

Bake for about 1 hour, or until golden brown. Remove from the heat and transfer to a serving plate.

Serve with cooked vegetables or fresh salad.

Nutrition information per serving: Kcal: 269, Protein: 25.3g, Carbs: 17.6g, Fats: 11.7g

48.   Eggplant Tomato Soup

Ingredients:

2 medium-sized eggplants, peeled and cubed

2 large tomatoes, peeled and diced

1 medium-sized red onion, finely chopped

2 tbsp of olive oil

1 tsp of salt

½ tsp of black pepper, ground

½ cup of sour cream

½ tsp of dried oregano, ground

Preparation:

Peel the eggplants and cut into small cubes. Set aside.

Preheat the oil in a large skillet over a medium-high temperature. Add onions and stir-fry for 3 minutes and then add eggplants. Stir well and cook for 5 minutes. Add diced tomatoes and stir well. Pour 1 cup of water and bring it to a boil, stirring occasionally.

Remove from the heat and set aside to cool. Transfer to a food processor and blend until nicely pureed. Return to the pot and add about 3 cups of water. Bring it to a boil and then stir in the sour cream and oregano. Cook until heated through and remove from the heat.

Serve warm.

Nutrition information per serving: Kcal: 277, Protein: 5.7g, Carbs: 28.1g, Fats: 18.2g

49. Creamy Beans

Ingredients:

1 lb of kidney beans, soaked and pre-cooked

1 medium-sized onion, finely chopped

1 tsp of cayenne pepper

3 tbsp of sour cream

¼ cup of fresh celery, finely chopped

2 tbsp of olive oil

1 tsp of salt

½ tsp of black pepper, ground

Preparation:

Soak the beans overnight. Rinse well under running water and place in a heavy-bottomed pot. Add 5 cups of water and bring it to a boil. Cook for 20 minutes, or until soften. Remove from the heat and drain. Set aside.

Preheat the oil in a heavy-bottomed pot over a medium-high temperature. Add onions and stir-fry until translucent. Add beans and 2 tablespoons of water. Stir well and cook for 5 minutes. Add sour cream, cayenne pepper, and celery. Cook for 3 more minutes.

Add water to adjust the thickness and cook for 2 more minutes, or until the mixture is nice and creamy.

Serve warm.

Nutrition information per serving: Kcal: 476, Protein: 26.3g, Carbs: 73.1g, Fats: 10.2g

50.   Chicken Thighs with Coriander and Lime

Ingredients:

1 lb of chicken thighs

2 large limes, juiced

1 tsp of lime zest, freshly grated

5 garlic cloves, finely chopped

½ cup of dry white wine

1 cup of chicken broth

1 tbsp of coriander, finely chopped

1 cup of couscous

¼ cup of olive oil

1 tsp of salt

¼ tsp of black pepper, ground

Preparation:

Preheat the oven to 375°F.

Wash the chicken thighs under cold running water. Pat dry with a kitchen paper and set aside. Rub the thighs with salt, cayenne, and pepper. Set aside to allow flavors to blend into the meat.

Preheat 1 tablespoon of oil in a large skillet over a medium-high temperature. Add chicken and cook for 5 minutes on each side, or until golden brown. Remove the chicken from the skillet and add wine. Reduce the heat to low and cook for 3 minutes, or until the mixture thickens. Add chicken broth and bring it to a boil. Add garlic, lime juice, and lime zest. Return the thighs to the skillet and sprinkle with coriander. Cook for 5 minutes and add few lime slices if you like. However, this is optional.

Transfer all on a large baking sheet and place it in the oven. Bake for about 35-40 minutes.

Meanwhile, combine the remaining oil, salt, and 2 ½ cups of water. Bring it to a boil and add couscous. Stir well and reduce the heat to low. Cook for 1 minute and then remove from the heat. Fluff with a fork and cover with a lid. Set aside.

Combine chicken thighs with couscous on a serving plate. Drizzle with some extra lime juice and serve immediately.

Enjoy!

Nutrition information per serving: Kcal: 429, Protein: 32.1g, Carbs: 31.6g, Fats: 17.4g

51.   Lima Beans and Spinach

Ingredients:

1 cup of lima beans, soaked overnight

1 cup of spinach

½ cup of fennel, chopped

1 medium-sized onion, chopped

¼ cup of chicken broth

1 tbsp of balsamic vinegar

1 tbsp of olive oil

1 tbsp of chives, finely chopped

½ tsp of black pepper, ground

½ tsp of salt

Preparation:

Soak the lima beans overnight. Drain and place in a deep pot. Add 3 cups of water and bring it to a boil. Cook for 10 minutes and remove from the heat. Drain well and set aside.

Preheat the oil in a medium skillet over a medium-high

temperature. Add onions and fennel. Simmer for 3 minutes, or until the onions translucent.

Add lima beans and chicken stock. Stir well and cook for 2 minutes and then add spinach. Reduce the heat to low and cover with a lid. Cook for 5 more minutes, or until spinach is wilted.

Stir in the balsamic vinegar and sprinkle with salt and pepper. Remove from the heat and transfer to a serving plate. Sprinkle with chives and enjoy!

Nutrition information per serving: Kcal: 189, Protein: 7.4g, Carbs: 23.6g, Fats: 8g

52. Sage Soup

Ingredients:

2 cups of fresh sage, roughly chopped

1 medium-sized onion, finely chopped

1 tbsp of all-purpose flour

1 cup of bone broth

1 tsp of cayenne pepper, ground

½ tsp of garlic powder

2 tbsp of olive oil

½ cup of sour cream

Preparation:

Wash the sage thoroughly under cold running water. Drain well and place in deep pot. Add enough water to cover and bring it to a boil. Cook for 1 minute and remove from the heat. Drain well and transfer to a food processor. Blend until finely chopped and set aside.

Preheat the oil in a large skillet over a medium-high temperature. Add onion and stir-fry for 3 minutes, or until translucent. Add flour, garlic, and ½ cup of water. Reduce the heat to low and simmer for 2 more minutes. Add broth and 1 cup of water. Bring it to a boil and then add sage. Cook for 15 minutes and then remove from the heat.

Stir in the sour cream and serve immediately.

Nutrition information per serving: Kcal: 203, Protein: 4.7g, Carbs: 16.8g, Fats: 15.5g

53.   Zucchini Roses in Cream

Ingredients:

1 large zucchini, cut into thin slices

1 cup of sour cream

½ cup of cream cheese

1 cup of fresh parsley, finely chopped

½ cup of spring onions, chopped

1 tsp of salt

1 tbsp of fresh dill, finely chopped

½ tsp of black pepper, ground

1 tbsp of olive oil

Preparation:

Wash the zucchini and cut into thin slices. Set aside.

In a large bowl, combine cheese, sour cream, parsley, dill, spring onions, pepper, and salt. Stir until well incorporated. Set aside.

Preheat the oil in a large frying pan over a medium-high temperature. Add zucchini slices and sprinkle with some salt. Cook for 2 minutes on each side and remove from the heat.

Now, roll the zucchini slices into rose shapes and tuck it in into the cream sauce. Garnish with parsley leaves and refrigerate for 20 minutes before serving.

Enjoy!

Nutrition information per serving: Kcal: 372, Protein: 7.8g, Carbs: 11.2g, Fats: 34.7g

54. Green Pepper Frittata

Ingredients:

4 large red bell peppers, chopped

½ cup of Feta cheese, crumbled

3 garlic cloves, crushed

1 tbsp of fresh parsley, finely chopped

2 tbsp of olive oil

3 large eggs

½ cup of Greek yogurt

2 tbsp of all-purpose flour

½ tsp of baking powder

¼ tsp of black pepper, ground

¼ tsp of salt

Preparation:

Preheat the oven to 375°F.

Wash the bell peppers and cut lengthwise in half. Remove the seeds and cut into small pieces. Set aside.

Preheat 1 tablespoon of olive oil in a large frying pan over a medium-high temperature. Add garlic and stir-fry for 1 minute and then add peppers. Cook for 3 minutes, stirring occasionally. Remove from the heat and set aside.

In a large bowl, combine eggs, yogurt, flour, and baking powder. Stir until well incorporated and set aside.

Grease a small baking dish with the remaining oil. Add bell peppers mixture and pour the egg mixture.

Place it in the oven and bake for 10 minutes, or until the top thickens. Remove from the oven and set aside to cool for a while before serving.

Nutrition information per serving: Kcal: 318, Protein: 15.6g, Carbs: 20.3g, Fats: 20.8g

55.   Tarragon Veal Roast

Ingredients:

2 lb of veal shoulder, tied

2 tbsp of olive oil

2 garlic clove, minced

2 large onions, finely chopped

2 tbsp of fresh parsley, finely chopped

1 tsp of dried thyme, ground

¼ tsp of cumin, ground

1 tsp of dried tarragon

1 tsp of sea salt

½ tsp of black pepper, freshly ground

Preparation:

Preheat the oven to 325°F.

Wash the meat under cold running water and pat dry with a kitchen paper. Set aside.

In a medium bowl, combine salt, pepper, and cumin. Stir well and rub over the meat. Set aside.

Preheat 1 tablespoon of olive oil in a large skillet over a medium-high temperature. Add onions and garlic and stir-fry for about 3-4 minutes, or until translucent. Add tarragon and reduce the heat to low. Cook for 10 minutes and remove from the heat.

Preheat the remaining oil in a large ovenproof pan over a medium-high temperature. Add meat and cook for about 10 minutes, or until browned on all sides. Now, add tarragon mixture and sprinkle with parsley and thyme.

Cover the pan with a lid and place it in the oven. Bake for about 25-30 minutes, or until tender.

Remove from the oven and skim fat from cooking juices. Cut the meat into ½ inch thick pieces and drizzle with the cooking juice.

Serve immediately.

Nutrition information per serving: Kcal: 551, Protein: 82.1g, Carbs: 8.1g, Fats: 19.3g

56.   Pineapple Banana Smoothie

Ingredients:

1 cup of pineapple, canned in juice

1 large banana, chopped

1 cup of Greek yogurt

1 tsp of vanilla extract

2 tbsp of lemon juice, freshly squeezed

Preparation:

Peel the banana cut into chunks. Transfer to a food processor or a blender. Add pineapple, yogurt, vanilla, and freshly squeezed lemon juice.

Blend until nicely creamy and transfer to serving glasses. Add some ice or refrigerate for 15 minutes before serving.

You can top with some fruit of your choice. For example, cherries are a great choice if you like. However, this is optional.

Enjoy!

Nutrition information per serving: Kcal: 186, Protein: 11.3g, Carbs: 30.9g, Fats: 2.4g

57. Spinach Tomato Salad with Garlic Vinaigrette

Ingredients:

2 large tomatoes, chopped

1 cup of fresh spinach, roughly chopped

1 large red bell pepper, chopped

1 small red onion, sliced

4 garlic cloves, finely chopped

1 tbsp of red wine vinegar

2 tbsp of olive oil

½ tsp of salt

½ tsp of black pepper, ground

Preparation:

Wash the tomatoes and cut into bite-sized pieces. Place it in a large bowl and set aside. Make sure to reserve the juice while cutting tomatoes.

Wash the spinach thoroughly under cold running water and roughly chop it. Add it to the bowl and set aside.

Wash the bell pepper and cut lengthwise in half. Remove the seeds and cut into small pieces. Set aside.

Peel the onion and slice into thin slices. Place in a small bowl and soak in salted water for 3 minutes to reduce the bitterness. When soaked, slightly drain and add it to the bowl.

In a small saucepan, combine garlic and 4 tablespoons of water. Bring it to a boil and reduce the heat to low. Simmer for 5 minutes until reduced liquid to 2 tablespoons. Remove from the heat and drain the garlic. Transfer to a small bowl and stir in the vinegar, olive oil, salt, and pepper. Stir until well combined and set aside for 15 minutes to allow flavors to meld.

Now, stir in the garlic dressing to a salad bowl. Toss until all well coat and serve immediately.

Nutrition information per serving: Kcal: 201, Protein: 3.5g, Carbs: 17.8g, Fats: 14.7g

58. Veal with Green Beans

Ingredients:

1 lb of lean veal, cut into bite-sized pieces

1 lb of green beans, cut into 1-inch pieces

3 tbsp of olive oil

1 medium-sized onion, finely chopped

2 garlic cloves, finely chopped

1 cup of bone broth

½ tsp of dried thyme, ground

½ tsp of salt

¼ tsp of black pepper, ground

Preparation:

Wash the meat under cold running water and pat dry with a kitchen paper. Cut into bite-sized pieces and set aside.

Using a large colander, rinse and drain the beans. Cut into 1-inch pieces and place in a large saucepan. Add 3 cups of water and bring it to a boil. Cook for 10 minutes and then remove from the heat. Drain well and set aside.

Preheat the oil in large saucepan over a medium-high temperature. Add onions and stir-fry for about 3-4 minutes, or until translucent. Add garlic and meat chops. Sprinkle with salt, pepper, and thyme. Cook for 7-10 minutes, or until the meat is browned. Stir occasionally.

Add broth and stir in the beans. Reduce the heat to low and cook for 5-7 minutes, stirring constantly. Remove from the heat and transfer to a serving plate.

Sprinkle with some fresh parsley. However, it's optional.

Nutrition information per serving: Kcal: 355, Protein: 35.1g, Carbs: 11.3g, Fats: 19.2g

59.   Grilled Marinated Mackerel

Ingredients:

1 lb of mackerel fillets

1 cup of brown rice

1 cup of olive oil

½ tsp of dried marjoram, ground

½ tsp of fresh rosemary, finely chopped

2 garlic cloves, crushed

¼ tsp of smoked paprika

2 tbsp of lemon juice, freshly squeezed

½ tsp of turmeric, ground

½ tsp of sea salt

½ tsp of black pepper, freshly ground

Preparation:

Wash the fillets thoroughly and pat dry with a kitchen paper. Set aside.

Place rice in a deep pot. Add 2 cups of water and bring it to a boil. Reduce the heat to low and stir in the turmeric. Cook for 15 minutes, or until the water almost evaporated. Remove from the heat and fluff with a fork. Set aside.

In a large bowl, combine oil, marjoram, rosemary, garlic, paprika, lemon juice, salt, and pepper. Mix until well incorporated and soak the fish in this marinade. Refrigerate for 30 minutes to allow flavors to penetrate into the fish.

Preheat the grill to a medium-high temperature. Place the fillets on a rack and grill for about 4-5 minutes on each side.

Remove from the grill and transfer to a serving plate. Add rice and serve immediately.

Nutrition information per serving: Kcal: 754, Protein: 41.1g, Carbs: 49.9g, Fats: 42.8g

60.   Mexican Pozole

Ingredients:

1 lb of lean beef, cut into cubes

1 cup of dried beans

1 cup of tomatoes, diced

1 tbsp of tomato paste

1 medium-sized onion, finely chopped

1 garlic clove, finely chopped

¼ cup of fresh cilantro, finely chopped

1 tbsp of olive oil

½ tsp of salt

¼ tsp of black pepper, freshly ground

Preparation:

Wash the meat under cold running water and pat dry with a kitchen paper. Cut into bite-sized cubes and place in a medium bowl. Rub the meat with salt and pepper and set aside.

Preheat the oil in a heavy-bottomed pot over a medium-high temperature. Add meat chops and cook for 10 minutes, or until nicely browned. Reduce the heat to low and add onions, garlic, and cilantro. Add water enough to cover all ingredients and bring it to a boil. Now, add tomatoes, tomato paste, and dried beans. Cover with a lid and cook for about 35-40 minutes, stirring occasionally. Add more water for the desired consistency. Remove from the heat and serve warm.

Nutrition information per serving: Kcal: 364, Protein: 47.8g, Carbs: 9.9g, Fats: 14.4g

61.   Chicken with Mushroom Sauce

Ingredients:

1 whole chicken, about 2 lbs

1 cup of button mushrooms, sliced

½ cup of shallots, finely chopped

3 garlic cloves, minced

½ cup of green olives, unpitted

½ cup of white wine

1 tsp of salt

½ tsp of black pepper, ground

Preparation:

Preheat the oven to 350°F.

Split the chicken down the backbone with a sharp heavy knife. Cut into two halves and turn the breast side up. Slightly press and flatten with the palm of your hand. Generously sprinkle with some salt and pepper.

Grease a large baking sheet and place the chicken. Place it in the oven and bake for about 40-45 minutes.

Meanwhile, combine mushrooms, shallots, garlic, olives, salt, and pepper. Stir until well incorporated. Remove the chicken from the oven and transfer to a plate. Add mushroom mixture and spread evenly on the baking sheet. Drizzle with wine. Now, return the chicken on top of the mixture and place again in the oven. Bake for about 40 minutes more and then remove from the oven.

Cut the chicken into serving pieces and spoon the mushrooms over it.

Serve warm.

Nutrition information per serving: Kcal: 396, Protein: 67.1g, Carbs: 6.1g, Fats: 7.5g

62.   Grapefruit Apple Juice

Ingredients:

1 large grapefruit, peeled

1 medium-sized apple, cored

1 medium-sized lemon, peeled

5 small radishes, trimmed and chopped

¼ tsp of ginger, ground

¼ tsp of cinnamon, ground

Preparation:

Peel the grapefruit and divide into wedges. Set aside.

Wash the apple and cut lengthwise in half. Remove the core and cut into bite-sized pieces. Set aside.

Peel the lemon and cut lengthwise in half. Set aside.

Wash the radishes and trim off the green parts. Cut into small pieces and set aside.

Now, combine grapefruit, apple, lemon, radishes, ginger, and cinnamon in a juicer and process until well juiced. Transfer to serving glasses and add 4 tablespoons of water. Stir well and add few ice cubes before serving.

Enjoy!

Nutrition information per serving: Kcal: 244, Protein: 3.5g, Carbs: 64.2g, Fats: 1g

63.   Creamy Chicken Tortillas

Ingredients:

1 lb of chicken breasts, skinless and boneless

½ cup of cheddar cheese

¼ cup of sour cream

1 large red bell pepper, chopped

¼ tsp of chili pepper, ground

¼ tsp of green pepper, ground

½ tsp of salt

1 tbsp of olive oil

5 whole wheat tortillas

Preparation:

Wash the chicken and pat dry with a kitchen paper. Cut into thin slices and set aside.

Wash the bell pepper and cut lengthwise in half. Remove the seeds and chop into small pieces. Set aside.

Preheat the oil in a large saucepan over a medium-high temperature. add chicken and sprinkle with some salt and pepper. Cook for 5-7 minutes, or until golden brown. Remove the chicken from the saucepan and add bell pepper. Cook for 3-4 minutes, or until tender. Sprinkle with green pepper, chili, and a pinch of salt. Stir well and then add chicken. Cook for 1 minute and reduce the heat to low. Stir in the sour cream and cheese.

Cook for 2 minutes and remove from the heat.

Spoon the mixture onto tortillas and roll. Serve immediately.

Nutrition information per serving: Kcal: 441, Protein: 34.7g, Carbs: 29.5g, Fats: 20.7g

64.   Strawberry Banana Oatmeal

Ingredients:

1 cup of fresh strawberries, chopped

1 medium-sized banana, sliced

1 tbsp of chia seeds

2 tbsp of lemon juice, freshly squeezed

1 cup of rolled oats

1 cup of milk

1 tbsp of honey, raw

Preparation:

In a medium pot, combine rolled oats and milk. Stir well and bring it to a boil. Remove from the heat and fluff with a fork. Set aside to soak for 10 minutes.

Meanwhile, wash the strawberries and cut into bite-sized pieces. Place in a medium bowl and set aside.

Peel the banana and cut into thin slices. Add it to the bowl with strawberries and drizzle with lemon juice. Set aside for 3 minutes to allow juice to meld in the fruits.

Now, stir in the strawberries and banana into the oatmeal. Top with chia seeds and refrigerate for 10 minutes before serving.

Enjoy!

Nutrition information per serving: Kcal: 405, Protein: 13.8g, Carbs: 66.9g, Fats: 10.5g

65.   Acorn Squash Cream Soup

Ingredients:

2 medium-sized acorn squash

4 cups of chicken broth

3 garlic cloves, finely chopped

3 tbsp of olive oil

2 tbsp of lime juice, freshly squeezed

1 medium-sized onion, roughly chopped

½ cup of sour cream

1 tsp of black pepper, ground

½ tsp of salt

Preparation:

Preheat the oven to 350°F.

Cut the squash lengthwise in half and scoop out the seeds. Place it on a large baking sheet and set aside.

Peel the onion and cut into large pieces. Spread evenly over the squash.

In a small bowl, combine olive oil and garlic. Drizzle over the squash. Place it in the oven and bake for about 40-45 minutes, or until nicely tender. Remove from the oven and allow it to cool completely.

Now, transfer all to a large saucepan and add the remaining ingredients.

Cover with a lid and cook for 15 minutes on a low temperature. Transfer to a food processor and blend until smooth and creamy.

Stir in the sour cream and reheat. Sprinkle with some more salt and pepper if you like. However, it's optional.

Serve warm.

Nutrition information per serving: Kcal: 294, Protein: 8g, Carbs: 28.9g, Fats: 18.2g

66.   Celery Pear Salad

Ingredients:

2 medium-sized celery stalks, chopped

2 large pears, cored and sliced

¼ cup of prunes, chopped

2 large oranges, peeled and wedged

½ cup of Greek yogurt

2 tbsp of lemon juice, freshly squeezed

½ tsp of salt

Preparation:

Wash the celery stalks and cut into bite-sized pieces. Set aside.

Wash the pears and cut lengthwise in half. Remove the core and cut into bite-sized pieces. Set aside.

Peel the oranges and divide into wedges. Set aside.

In a small bowl, combine lemon juice, greek yogurt, and salt. Stir until well incorporated and set aside to allow flavors to blend.

In a large salad bowl, combine celery, pears, oranges, and prunes. Stir once and then drizzle with previously prepared dressing.

Toss well to coat and refrigerate for 15 minutes before serving.

Enjoy!

Nutrition information per serving: Kcal: 306, Protein: 8.4g, Carbs: 70.6g, Fats: 1.8g

67.   Shrimp Stuffed Portobello

Ingredients:

6 Portobello mushrooms

4 oz of shrimps, cleaned

2 tbsp of Parmesan cheese, grated

1 tsp of smoked paprika, ground

1 garlic clove, minced

1 tbsp of olive oil

½ tsp of Worcestershire sauce

½ tsp of salt

Preparation:

Preheat the oven to 350°F.

Wash the mushrooms and remove the stems. Place them on a large baking sheet with bottom up. Set aside.

Clean and devein the shrimps. Wash thoroughly under cold running water and pat dry with a kitchen paper. Place in a medium bowl and set aside.

Finely chop the garlic and add it to the shrimps. Sprinkle with smoked paprika and stir well to coat. Set aside.

Preheat the oil in a medium saucepan over a medium-high temperature. Add shrimp mixture and cook for about 4-5 minutes, stirring occasionally. Remove from the heat and stuff the prepared mushrooms with shrimps.

Sprinkle with Parmesan and place it in the oven. Bake for 5 minutes, or until set.

Remove from the heat and serve immediately.

Enjoy!

Nutrition information per serving: Kcal: 239, Protein: 26.7g, Carbs: 11.7g, Fats: 11.1g

68.   Crispy Tilapia

Ingredients:

1 lb of tilapia fillets

1 tbsp of fresh basil, finely chopped

1 cup of cornmeal

2 tbsp of all-purpose flour

2 large eggs

4 tbsp of Parmesan cheese, grated

½ tsp of salt

¼ tsp of black pepper, ground

2 tbsp of lemon juice, freshly squeezed

1tbsp of olive oil

Preparation:

Preheat the oven to 450°F. Grease a large baking sheet with some olive oil and set aside.

Wash the fillets under cold water and pat dry with a kitchen paper. Cut into thin slices and set aside.

In a large mixing bowl, combine cornmeal, flour, and cheese, Stir well until combine and set aside.

Whisk the eggs in a medium bowl until foamy. Set aside.

Now, coat fillets in the eggs, then in flour mixture. Spread evenly on a previously prepared sheet and place it in the oven.

Bake for about 15-20 minutes, or until nicely crisp. Remove from the heat and serve with some sweet potato puree or steamed greens.

Nutrition information per serving: Kcal: 662, Protein: 63.4g, Carbs: 54.8g, Fats: 22.4g

69.   Mango Apricot Porridge

Ingredients:

2 large mangos, peeled and chunked

2 medium-sized apricots, finely chopped

½ cup of skim milk

½ cup of cream

1 tbsp of honey

2 tbsp of almonds

1 tbsp of orange juice, freshly squeezed

Preparation:

Peel the mangos and cut into small chunks. Place it in a food processor and add orange juice and honey. Blend until nicely combined and transfer to a medium bowl. Set aside.

Wash the apricots and cut lengthwise in half. Remove the pits and finely chop it. Add it to the bowl with mango along with milk and cream. Stir all well and top with almonds.

Refrigerate for 15 minutes before serving and enjoy!

Nutrition information per serving: Kcal: 349, Protein: 7.1g, Carbs: 69.4g, Fats: 7.9g

JUICES

1.   Celery Grapefruit Juice

Ingredients:

1 cup of celery, chopped

1 whole grapefruit, peeled

2 large carrots, chunked

1 small Golden Delicious apple, cored and chopped

¼ tsp of cinnamon, ground

Preparation:

Wash the celery and cut into small pieces. Fill the measuring cup and reserve the rest in the refrigerator.

Peel the grapefruit and divide into wedges. Cut each wedge in half and set aside.

Wash and peel the carrots. Cut into small chunks and set aside.

Wash the apple and cut lengthwise in half. Remove the core and cut into bite-sized pieces. Set aside.

Now, combine carrots, celery, grapefruit, and apple in a juicer and process until well juiced. Transfer to a serving glass and stir in the cinnamon.

Add some crushed ice and serve immediately.

Nutritional information per serving: Kcal: 203, Protein: 4.3g, Carbs: 60.6g, Fats: 1.1g

2.   Basil Cucumber Juice

Ingredients:

1 cup of basil, torn

1 cup of cucumber, sliced

1 medium-sized artichoke, chopped

1 whole lime, peeled

2 oz of water

Preparation:

Wash the basil thoroughly under cold running water. Drain and torn into small pieces. Set aside.

Wash the cucumber and cut into thin slices. Fill the measuring cup and reserve the rest in the refrigerator.

Trim off the outer leaves of the artichoke. Wash it and chop into small pieces. Set aside.

Peel the lime and cut lengthwise in half. Set aside.

Now, combine artichoke, basil, cucumber, and lime in a juicer and process until juiced. Transfer to a serving glass and stir in the water.

Refrigerate for 5 minutes before serving.

Nutrition information per serving: Kcal: 53, Protein: 5.5g, Carbs: 19.6g, Fats: 0.4g

3.   Asparagus Collard Green Juice

Ingredients:

1 medium-sized tomato, chopped

1 cup of asparagus, trimmed and chopped

1 cup of collard greens, torn

1 cup of spinach, torn

¼ tsp salt

1 rosemary sprig

Preparation:

Wash the asparagus and trim off the woody ends. Cut into small pieces and fill the measuring cup. Set aside.

Combine collard greens and spinach in a large colander. Wash under cold running water and drain. Torn into small pieces and set aside.

Wash the tomato and place it in a small bowl. Cut into small pieces and reserve the tomato juice while cutting. Set aside.

Now, combine asparagus, collard greens, tomato, and spinach in a juicer and process until juiced. Transfer to a serving glass and stir in the reserve tomato juice and salt. Sprinkle with rosemary.

You can add some basil for some extra taste, but it's optional.

Serve immediately.

Nutritional information per serving: Kcal: 66, Protein: 11.2g, Carbs: 19.6g, Fats: 1.5g

4.   Kiwi Apple Juice

Ingredients:

1 whole kiwi, peeled

1 small Grany Smith's apple, cored

1 cup of mango, chopped

1 small ginger knob, peeled

2 oz of coconut water

Preparation:

Peel the kiwi and cut lengthwise in half. Set aside.

Wash the apple and cut lengthwise in half. Remove the core and cut into small pieces. Set aside.

Peel the mango and cut into small pieces. Fill the measuring cup and reserve the rest for later.

Peel the ginger knob and cut into small pieces. Set aside.

Now, combine mango, kiwi, apple, and ginger in a juicer and process until juiced. Transfer to a serving glass and stir in the coconut water. Add some crushed ice and serve immediately.

Enjoy!

Nutrition information per serving: Kcal: 196, Protein: 2.8g, Carbs: 55.5g, Fats: 1.3g

5.   Celery Plum Juice

Ingredients:

1 cup of celery, chopped

1 whole plum, pitted and chopped

1 small Golden Delicious apple, cored

1 cup of cherries

¼ tsp of cinnamon, ground

2 tbsp of coconut water

Preparation:

Wash and trim off the celery. Chop into small pieces and set aside.

Wash the plum and cut in half. Remove the pit and chop into small pieces. Set aside.

Wash the apple and cut lengthwise in half. Remove the core and cut into bite-sized pieces. Set aside.

Wash the cherries using a colander. Drain and cut each in half. Remove the pits and set aside.

Now, combine celery, plum, apple, cherries, in a juicer and process until juiced. Transfer to a serving glass and stir in the cinnamon and coconut water.

Add some crushed ice and serve immediately.

Nutritional information per serving: Kcal: 182, Protein: 3.1g, Carbs: 52.7g, Fats: 0.8g

6.   Squash Zucchini Juice

Ingredients:

1 cup of butternut squash, chopped

1 cup of crookneck squash, chopped

1 large zucchini

1 cup of pumpkin, chopped

1 large carrot

¼ tsp of nutmeg, ground

¼ tsp of salt

2 oz of water

Preparation:

Peel the butternut squash and remove the seeds using a spoon. Cut into small cubes and reserve the rest of the squash for some other recipe. Wrap in a plastic foil and refrigerate.

Wash the crookneck squash and cut in half. Scoop out the seeds using a spoon. Cut into small chunks and set aside. Reserve the rest for another juice.

Peel the zucchini and cut in lengthwise in half. Scrap out the seeds and cut into chunks. Set aside.

Peel the pumpkin and cut in half. Scoop out the seeds using a spoon. Cut one large wedge and peel it. Cut into small chunks and set aside. Reserve the rest for later.

Wash the carrot and cut into thick slices. Set aside.

Now, process butternut squash, crookneck squash, zucchini, pumpkin, and carrot in a juicer.

Transfer to serving glasses and stir in the Himalayan salt and water. Refrigerate for 5 minutes before serving.

Enjoy!

Nutritional information per serving: Kcal: 163, Protein: 8.4g, Carbs: 45.8g, Fats: 1.8g

7.   Carrot Pepper Juice

Ingredients:

1 large carrot

1 large red bell pepper

1 cup of cauliflower, chopped

1 large orange

1 cup of fresh kale, torn

¼ tsp of Himalayan salt

3 oz of water

Preparation:

Wash the carrot and cut into thick slices. Set aside.

Wash the red bell pepper and cut in half. Remove the seeds and cut in small pieces. Set aside.

Trim off the outer leaves of a cauliflower. Wash it and cut into small pieces and fill the measuring cup. Reserve the rest in the refrigerator.

Peel the orange and divide into wedges. Set aside.

Wash the kale thoroughly and torn with hands. Set aside.

Now, process carrot, red bell pepper, cauliflower, orange, and kale in a juicer. Transfer to serving glasses and stir in the salt and water.

Refrigerate for 5 minutes before serving.

Enjoy!

Nutritional information per serving: Kcal: 169, Protein: 8.9g, Carbs: 49.6g, Fats: 1.8g

8.   Apple Cucumber Juice

Ingredients:

1 large Granny Smith apple

1 large cucumber

1 large fennel

1 rosemary sprig

¼ tsp of Himalayan salt

2 oz of water

Preparation:

Wash the apple and remove the core. Cut into bite-sized pieces and set aside.

Wash the cucumber and cut into thick pieces. Set aside.

Wash the fennel bulb and trim off the wilted outer layers. Cut into small chunks and set aside.

Now, process fennel, apple, and cucumber in a juicer. Transfer to serving glasses and stir in the Himalayan salt and water. Sprinkle with rosemary and refrigerate for 10 minutes before serving.

Enjoy!

Nutritional information per serving: Kcal: 179, Protein: 5.7g, Carbs: 56g, Fats: 1.2g

9. Carrot Apple Juice

Ingredients:

3 large carrots

1 large green apple, cored

1 large orange

1 cup of watermelon, diced

1 cup of green grapes

1 small ginger root knob, 1-inch

Preparation:

Wash the carrots and cut into thick slices. Set aside.

Wash the apple and remove the core. Cut into bite-sized pieces and set aside.

Peel the orange and divide into wedges. Set aside.

Cut the watermelon lengthwise. For one cup, you will need about 1 large wedge. Peel and cut into chunks. Remove the seeds and set aside. Reserve the rest of the melon for some other juices.

Wash the grapes under cold running water. Drain and set aside.

Peel the ginger root knob and set aside.

Now, combine carrots, apple, orange, watermelon, grapes, and ginger in a juicer and process until juiced.

Transfer to serving glasses and add some ice before serving.

Enjoy!

Nutritional information per serving: Kcal: 335, Protein: 6.2g, Carbs: 98g, Fats: 1.7g

10. Leek Lime Juice

Ingredients:

1 whole leek, chopped

1 whole lime, peeled

1 large orange, peeled

1 small green apple, cored

Preparation:

Wash the leek and chop into small pieces. Set aside.

Peel the lemon and lime. Cut each fruit lengthwise in half and set aside.

Peel the orange and divide into wedges. Cut each wedge in half and set aside.

Wash the apple and cut in half. Remove the core and cut into small pieces. Set aside.

Now, combine lemon, leek, lime, orange, and apple in a juicer and process until juiced. Transfer to a serving glass and refrigerate for 15 minutes before serving.

Enjoy!

Nutrition information per serving: Kcal: 205, Protein: 4.5g, Carbs: 62.9g, Fats: 0.9g

11.   Pineapple Raspberry Juice

Ingredients:

1 cup of pineapple chunks

1 cup of raspberries

1 large mango

1 large orange

2 oz of coconut water

Preparation:

Cut the top of a pineapple and peel it using a sharp knife. Cut into small chunks. Reserve the rest of the pineapple in a refrigerator.

Place the raspberries in a colander and wash under cold running water. Drain and set aside.

Wash the mango and cut into bite-sized pieces. Set aside.

Peel the orange and divide into wedges. Set aside.

Now, combine, pineapple, raspberries, mango, and orange in a juicer and process until juiced. Transfer to serving glasses and stir in the coconut water.

Add some ice and serve immediately!

Nutritional information per serving: Kcal: 353, Protein: 6.8, Carbs: 108g, Fats: 2.5g

12.   Blackberry Kiwi Juice

Ingredients:

1 cup of blackberries

2 whole kiwis, peeled

1 cup of cantaloupe, chopped

1 small green apple, cored

¼ tsp of ginger, ground

Preparation:

Place the blackberries in a colander. Rinse well under cold running water and drain. Set aside.

Peel the kiwi and cut in half. Set aside.

Cut the cantaloupe in half. Scrape out the seeds and cut one one large wedge. Peel and chop into small pieces. Wrap the rest in a plastic foil and refrigerate for later.

Wash the apple and cut lengthwise in half. Remove the core and cut into bite-sized pieces. Set aside.

Now, combine cantaloupe, blackberries, kiwi, and apple in a juicer and process until juiced. Transfer to a serving glass and stir in the ginger.

Add few ice cubes and serve immediately.

Nutritional information per serving: Kcal: 181, Protein: 4.7g, Carbs: 56.3g, Fats: 1.6g

13.   Cucumber Strawberry Juice

Ingredients:

1 cup of cucumber, sliced

1 cup of strawberries, chopped

1 cup of blueberries

1 cup of fresh mint, torn

1 large carrot, sliced

¼ tsp of cinnamon, ground

Preparation:

Wash the cucumber and cut into thin slices. Fill the measuring cup and reserve the rest in the refrigerator.

Wash the strawberries and remove the stems. Chop into small pieces and set aside.

Wash the blueberries using a small colander. Drain and set aside.

Wash the mint thoroughly under cold running water. Drain and torn into small pieces. Set aside.

Wash and peel the carrot. Cut into thin slices and set aside.

Now, combine cucumber, strawberries, blueberries, mint, and carrot in a juicer. Process until well juiced.

Transfer to a serving glass and stir in the cinnamon. Add some crushed ice and serve immediately!

Nutrition information per serving: Kcal: 141, Protein: 4g, Carbs: 45g, Fats: 1.3g

14.   Honeydew Melon Watercress Juice

Ingredients:

1 large honeydew melon wedge

1 cup of watercress, torn

1 large artichoke

1 large green apple, cored

1 cup of mustard greens, torn

2 oz of water

¼ tsp of agave nectar

Preparation:

Cut the honeydew melon lengthwise in half. Scoop out the seeds using a spoon. Cut one large wedge and peel it. Cut into small chunks and place in a bowl. Wrap the rest of the melon in a plastic foil and refrigerate.

Combine watercress and mustard greens in a colander and wash under cold running water. Drain and set aside.

Trim off the outer leaves of the artichoke using a sharp knife. Cut into bite-sized pieces and set aside.

Wash the apple and remove the core. Cut into bite-sized pieces and set aside.

Now, process honeydew melon, watercress, artichoke, apple, and mustard greens in a juicer. Transfer to serving glasses and stir in the water and agave nectar.

Add some ice and serve immediately.

Nutritional information per serving: Kcal: 261, Protein: 9.4g, Carbs: 79.6g, Fats: 1.1g

15. Kale Orange Juice

Ingredients:

1 cup of kale, torn

1 large orange, peeled

1 cup of pineapple, chunked

1 cup of mango, chopped

1 small ginger knob, chopped

Preparation:

Wash the kale thoroughly under cold running water. Drain and torn into small pieces. Set aside.

Peel the orange and divide into wedges. Cut each wedge in half and set aside.

Using a sharp paring knife, cut the top of the pineapple. Gently remove all hard skin and cut it into small chunks. Fill the measuring cup and reserve the rest for later.

Peel the mango and chop into small pieces. Fill the measuring cup and reserve the rest for later. Set aside.

Peel the ginger knob and cut into small pieces. Set aside.

Now, combine pineapple, mango, kale, orange, and ginger in a juicer and process until juiced. Transfer to a serving glass and refrigerate for 15 minutes before serving.

Enjoy!

Nutrition information per serving: Kcal: 258, Protein: 6.9g, Carbs: 74.9g, Fats: 1.7g

16.   Tomato Basil Juice

Ingredients:

2 medium-sized Roma tomatoes, chopped

1 cup of fresh basil, torn

1 cup of pumpkin, cubed

1 large cucumber

¼ tsp of dried oregano

½ tsp of sea salt

2 oz of water

Preparation:

Wash the tomatoes and place them in a bowl. Cut into quarters and reserve the juice while cutting. Set aside.

Wash the basil thoroughly under cold running water. Torn with hands and set aside.

Peel the pumpkin and cut in half. Scoop out the seeds using a spoon. Cut one large wedge and peel it. Cut into small chunks and set aside. Reserve the rest for later.

Wash the cucumber and cut into thick slices. Set aside.

Now, process tomatoes, basil, pumpkin, and cucumber in a juicer. Transfer to serving glasses and stir in the oregano, salt, water, and reserved tomato juice.

Refrigerate for 5 minutes before serving.

Enjoy!

Nutritional information per serving: Kcal: 87, Protein: 4.9g, Carbs: 23.9g, Fats: 0.9g

17.   Peach Plum Juice

Ingredients:

1 large peach, chopped

1 whole plum, chopped

1 cup of mango, chopped

1 small Red Delicious apple, cored

1 oz of coconut water

Preparation:

Wash the peach and cut lengthwise in half. Remove the pit and cut into small pieces. Set aside.

Wash the plum and cut in half. Remove the pit and chop into small pieces. Set aside.

Peel the mango and cut into small cubes. Fill the measuring cup and reserve the rest for later.

Wash the apple cut lengthwise in half. Remove the core and chop into small pieces. Set aside.

Now, combine peach, plum, mango and apple in a juicer and process until juiced. Transfer to a serving glass and stir in the coconut water.

Add some ice and serve immediately.

Nutritional information per serving: Kcal: 252, Protein: 3.8g, Carbs: 71.1g, Fats: 1.6g

18.   Leek Beet Green Juice

Ingredients:

2 large leeks, chopped

1 cup of beet greens, torn

1 cup of broccoli

1 cup of arugula, torn

1 cup of collard greens, torn

1 large cucumber

1 large lime

A handful of spinach, torn

Preparation:

Wash the leeks and cut into small pieces. Set aside.

Combine arugula, beet greens, collard greens, and spinach in a colander. Wash under cold running water and torn with hands.

Wash the broccoli and cut into small chunks. Set aside.

Wash the cucumber and cut into thick slices. Set aside.

Peel the lime and cut lengthwise in half. Set aside.

Now, process arugula, beet greens, collard greens, spinach, leeks, broccoli, cucumber, and lime in a juicer. Transfer to serving glasses and refrigerate for 30 minutes before serving.

Enjoy!

Nutritional information per serving: Kcal: 194, Protein: 13.1g, Carbs: 55.7g, Fats: 1.8g

19.   Tomato Onion Juice

Ingredients:

1 medium-sized tomato, chopped

½ cup of spring onions, chopped

1 cup of cauliflower, chopped

½ cup of basil, torn

1 cup of cucumber, sliced

1 oz of water

Preparation:

Wash the tomato and place in a small bowl. Chop into small pieces and reserve the tomato juice while cutting. Set aside.

Wash the spring onions and basil. Chop into small pieces. Set aside.

Trim off the outer leaves of the cauliflower. Wash it and cut into small pieces. Fill the measuring cup and reserve the rest for later. Set aside.

Wash the cucumber and cut into thin slices. Fill the measuring cup and reserve the rest for later. Set aside.

Now, combine cauliflower, tomato, spring onions, basil, and cucumber in a juicer and process until well juiced. Transfer to a serving glass and stir in the water.

Serve cold.

Nutrition information per serving: Kcal: 51, Protein: 4.4g, Carbs: 13.9g, Fats: 0.7g

20. Blueberry Zucchini Juice

Ingredients:

1 cup of blueberries

1 medium-sized zucchini, sliced

2 cups of raspberries

1 small ginger knob, peeled

1 oz of coconut water

Preparation:

Combine raspberries and blueberries in a large colander. Rinse well under cold running water. Drain and set aside.

Wash the zucchini and cut into thin slices. Set aside.

Peel the ginger knob and cut into small pieces. Set aside.

Now, combine raspberries, blueberries, zucchini, and ginger in a juicer and process until juiced. Transfer to a serving glass and stir in the coconut water.

Add crushed ice or refrigerate for 15 minutes before serving.

Enjoy!

Nutritional information per serving: Kcal: 164, Protein: 6.5g, Carbs: 58g, Fats: 2.7g

21.   Swiss Chard Cauliflower Juice

Ingredients:

2 cups of Swiss chard

1 cup of cauliflower, chopped

3 large carrots, sliced

1 large lime, peeled

1 large orange, peeled

1 oz of water

Preparation:

Wash the Swiss chard thoroughly and torn with hands. Set aside.

Trim off the outer leaves of cauliflower. Wash it and cut into small pieces. Fill the measuring cup and reserve the rest in the refrigerator.

Wash the carrots and cut into thick slices. Set aside.

Peel the lime and cut lengthwise in half. Set aside.

Peel the orange and divide into wedges. Set aside.

Now, process carrots, Swiss chard, cauliflower, lime, and orange in a juicer. Transfer to serving glasses and stir in the water.

Add some ice and serve immediately.

Enjoy!

Nutritional information per serving: Kcal: 173, Protein: 7.3g, Carbs: 54g, Fats: 1.2g

22.   Raspberry Lemon Juice

Ingredients:

1 cup of raspberries

1 large lemon

1 large grapefruit

1 large lime

1 medium-sized yellow apple, cored

4oz of coconut water

Preparation:

Place the raspberries in a colander and wash under cold running water. Drain and set aside.

Peel the lemon and lime. Cut lengthwise in half and set aside.

Peel the grapefruit and divide into wedges. Set aside.

Wash the apple and remove the core. Cut into bite-sized pieces and set aside.

Now combine grapefruit, raspberries, lemon, lime, and apple in a juicer and process until juiced. Transfer to serving glasses and stir in the coconut water.

Add some ice and serve immediately.

Nutritional information per serving: Kcal: 240, Protein: 4.6g, Carbs: 76g, Fats: 1.6g

23.   Orange Spinach Juice

Ingredients:

1 large orange, peeled

½ cup of spinach, torn

1 cup of pineapple, chunked

3 Brussels sprouts, halved

Preparation:

Peel the orange and divide into wedges. Cut each wedge in half and set aside.

Wash the spinach thoroughly under cold running water and torn with hands. Set aside.

Using a sharp paring knife, cut the top of the pineapple. Gently remove all hard skin and slice it into thin slices. Fill the measuring cup and reserve the rest for later.

Wash the Brussels sprouts and trim off the wilted leaves. Cut each in half and set aside.

Now, combine orange, spinach, pineapple, and Brussels sprouts in a juicer and process until well juiced. Transfer to a serving glass and refrigerate for 15 minutes before serving.

Enjoy!

Nutrition information per serving: Kcal: 172, Protein: 7.9g, Carbs: 52.7g, Fats: 1.1g

24. Apple Ginger Juice

Ingredients:

1 small Golden Delicious apple, cored

¼ tsp of ginger, ground

1 cup of spinach, chopped

1 medium-sized wedge of honeydew melon

1 cup of raspberries

Preparation:

Wash the apple and cut lengthwise in half. Remove the core and cut into bite-sized pieces. Set aside.

Wash the spinach thoroughly under cold running water. Drain and chop into small pieces. Set aside.

Cut melon lengthwise in half. Scoop out the seeds and then wash the melon. Cut one wedge and peel it. Cut into bite-sized pieces and set aside. Reserve the rest in the refrigerator.

Place the raspberries in a colander and rinse well under cold running water. Drain and set aside.

Now, combine spinach, melon, raspberries, and apple in a juicer and process until juiced. Transfer to a serving glass and stir in the ginger. Add some ice before serving.

Enjoy!

Nutritional information per serving: Kcal: 142, Protein: 4.5g, Carbs: 46.1g, Fats: 1.4g

25. Pomegranate Orange Juice

Ingredients:

1 cup of pomegranate seeds

1 medium-sized orange, wedged

1 large pear, chopped

3 whole apricots, pitted

¼ tsp of cinnamon, ground

Preparation:

Cut the top of the pomegranate fruit using a sharp paring knife. Slice down to each of the white membranes inside of the fruit. Pop the seeds into a measuring cup and set aside.

Peel the orange and divide into wedges. Cut each wedge in half and set aside.

Wash the pear and cut lengthwise in half. Cut into bite-sized pieces and set aside.

Wash the apricots and cut each in half. Remove the pit and cut into small pieces. Set aside.

Now, combine pear, apricots, pomegranate seeds, and orange in a juicer. Process until well juiced. Transfer to a serving glass and stir in the cinnamon.

Refrigerate for 5 minutes before serving.

Nutrition information per serving: Kcal: 253, Protein: 4.9g, Carbs: 78.3g, Fats: 1.9g

26.   Celery Apple Juice

Ingredients:

1 cup of celery, chopped

1 medium-sized apple, cored

1 cup of sweet potatoes, cubed

1 medium-sized orange, peeled

1 tbsp of fresh mint, torn

Preparation:

Wash the celery and cut into bite-sized pieces. Set aside.

Wash the apple and cut lengthwise in half. Remove the core and cut into bite-sized pieces. Set aside.

Peel the sweet potato and cut into small cubes. Fill the measuring cup and reserve the rest for later. Set aside.

Peel the orange and divide into wedges. Cut each wedge in half and set aside.

Now, combine sweet potatoes, celery, apple, and orange in a juicer. Process until well juiced. Transfer to a serving glass and sprinkle with mint.

Add some crushed ice and serve immediately.

Nutrition information per serving: Kcal: 236, Protein: 4.7g, Carbs: 67.8g, Fats: 0.7g

27.   Artichoke Cucumber Juice

Ingredients:

1 large artichoke, chopped

1 cup of cucumber, sliced

2 cups of Brussels sprouts, halved

¼ tsp of turmeric, ground

¼ tsp of ginger, ground

2 oz of water

Preparation:

Trim off the outer leaves of the artichoke. Cut into small pieces and set aside.

Wash the cucumber and cut into thin slices. Fill the measuring cup and reserve the rest in the refrigerator.

Wash the Brussels sprouts and trim off the outer layers. Cut each sprout in half and fill the measuring cups. Set aside.

Now, combine Brussels sprouts, artichoke, and cucumber in a juicer and process until well juiced. Transfer to a serving glass and stir in the ginger, turmeric, and water.

Refrigerate for 15 minutes before serving.

Enjoy!

Nutritional information per serving: Kcal: 98, Protein: 11.6g, Carbs: 34.7g, Fats: 0.8g

28.   Banana Strawberry Juice

Ingredients:

1 large banana, sliced

½ cup of strawberries, chopped

1 cup of avocado, chunked

1 cup of red leaf lettuce, shredded

1 small Red Delicious apple, cored

¼ tsp of cinnamon, ground

Preparation:

Peel the banana and chop into small pieces. Set aside.

Wash the strawberries and remove the stems. Cut into bite-sized pieces and fill the measuring cup. Set aside.

Peel the avocado and cut lengthwise in half. Remove the pit and chop into small pieces. Set aside.

Wash the lettuce thoroughly under cold running water. Drain and chop into small pieces. Set aside.

Now, combine avocado, lettuce, banana, and strawberries in a juicer and process until juiced. Transfer to a serving glass and stir in the cinnamon.

Add some ice and serve immediately.

Enjoy!

Nutritional information per serving: Kcal: 405, Protein: 5.7g, Carbs: 72.2g, Fats: 23.1g

29.   Basil Cucumber Juice

Ingredients:

1 cup of fresh basil, torn

1 cup of cucumber, sliced

1 cup of celery, chopped

1 whole lime, peeled

1 medium-sized apple, cored

Preparation:

Wash the basil thoroughly under cold running water. Drain and torn into small pieces. Set aside.

Wash the cucumber and cut into thin slices. Fill the measuring cup and reserve the rest for later. Set aside.

Wash the celery and cut into small pieces. Set aside.

Peel the lime and cut lengthwise in half. Set aside.

Wash the apple and cut lengthwise in half. Remove the core and cut into bite-sized pieces. Set aside.

Now, combine celery, basil, cucumber, lime, and apple in a juicer and process until well juiced. Transfer to a serving glass and add some crushed ice.

Serve immediately.

Nutritional information per serving: Kcal: 109, Protein: 2.7g, Carbs: 31.9g, Fats: 0.7g

30.   Orange Cantaloupe Juice

Ingredients:

1 large orange

1 cup of cantaloupe

1 cup of strawberries

1 large carrot

2 oz of water

Preparation:

Peel the orange and divide into wedges. Set aside.

Cut the cantaloupe in half. Scoop out the seeds. Cut two wedges and peel them. Chop into chunks and set aside. Reserve the rest of the cantaloupe in a refrigerator.

Wash the strawberries under cold running water. Drain and cut in half. Set aside.

Wash the carrot and cut into thick slices. Set aside.

Now, combine strawberries, orange, cantaloupe, and carrot in a juicer and process until juiced.

Transfer to serving glasses and stir in the water. Add some ice and serve immediately.

Nutritional information per serving: Kcal: 177, Protein: 4.9g, Carbs: 55g, Fats: 1.2g

31.   Apple Pomegranate Juice

Ingredients:

1 large red apple, cored

1 cup of pomegranate seeds

2 large beets, trimmed

1 large cucumber

1 small ginger knob, 1-inch

Preparation:

Wash the apple and remove the core. Cut into bite-sized pieces and set aside.

Cut the top of the pomegranate fruit using a sharp knife. Slice down to each of the white membranes inside of the fruit. Pop the seeds into a medium bowl.

Wash the beets and trim off the green parts. Cut into small pieces and set aside.

Wash the cucumber and cut into thick slices. Set aside.

Peel the ginger knob and set aside.

Now, process beets, apple, pomegranate seeds, cucumber and ginger knob in a juicer. Transfer to serving glasses and add some ice. You can stir in one tablespoon of honey, but this is optional.

Serve immediately.

Nutritional information per serving: Kcal: 285, Protein: 8g, Carbs: 81.6g, Fats: 2.2g

32.   Collard Green Cucumber Juice

Ingredients:

1 cup of collard greens, chopped

1 cup of cucumber, sliced

1 whole fennel bulb, chopped

1 whole lemon, peeled

1 oz of water

¼ tsp of cayenne pepper, ground

Preparation:

Rinse the collard greens under cold running water. Drain and chop into small pieces. Set aside.

Wash the cucumber and cut into thin slices. Fill the measuring cup and reserve the rest for later. Set aside.

Trim off the fennel bulb and remove the green parts. Wash the bulb and cut into small pieces. Set aside.

Peel the lemon and cut lengthwise in half. Set aside.

Now, combine fennel, collard greens, cucumber, and lemon in a juicer and process until juiced. Transfer to a serving glass and stir in the water and cayenne pepper.

Refrigerate for 20 minutes before serving.

Enjoy!

Nutritional information per serving: Kcal: 68, Protein: 4.9g, Carbs: 26.3g, Fats: 0.9g

33.   Apple Strawberry Juice

Ingredients:

1 small green apple, cored

1 cup of strawberries, chopped

1 cup of cherries, pitted

2 whole plums, pitted and chopped

1 tbsp of coconut water

¼ tsp of ginger, ground

Preparation:

Wash the apple and cut lengthwise in half. Remove the core and cut into small pieces. Set aside.

Wash the strawberries and remove the stems. Cut into small pieces and fill the measuring cup. Reserve the rest for later. Set aside.

Wash the cherries thoroughly using a large colander. Drain and cut each in half. Remove the pits and cut into small pieces. Set aside.

Wash the plums and cut in half. Remove the pits and cut into small bite-sized pieces. Set aside.

Now, combine apple, strawberries, cherries, and plums in a juicer and process until juiced. Transfer to a serving glass and stir in the coconut water and ginger.

Add some crushed ice and serve immediately.

Nutritional information per serving: Kcal: 236, Protein: 4.2g, Carbs: 70.3g, Fats: 1.3g

34.   Cabbage Avocado Juice

Ingredients:

1 cup of green cabbage, torn

1 cup of avocado, cubed

1 large artichoke, chopped

1 cup of fresh spinach, torn

¼ tsp of turmeric, ground

Preparation:

Combine spinach and cabbage in a large colander. Wash thoroughly under cold running water. Drain and torn into small pieces. Set aside.

Peel the avocado and cut lengthwise in half. Remove the pit and cut into small cubes. Fill the measuring cup and reserve the rest in the refrigerator.

Trim off the outer layers of the artichoke using a sharp paring knife. Cut into bite-sized pieces and set aside.

Now, combine artichoke, spinach, cabbage, and avocado in a juicer and process until juiced. Transfer to a serving glass and stir in the turmeric.

Refrigerate for 10 minutes before serving.

Nutritional information per serving: Kcal: 282, Protein: 15.4g, Carbs: 42.6g, Fats: 23.2g

35.   Avocado Cantaloupe Juice

Ingredients:

1 cup of avocado chunks

1 cup of cantaloupe, chopped

3 cups of celery, chopped

1 cup of fresh basil, torn

1 cup of cucumber, sliced

2 oz of water

Preparation:

Peel the avocado and cut in half. Remove the pit and cut into chunks. Fill the measuring cup and refrigerate the rest for some other juice.

Cut the cantaloupe in half. Scoop out the seeds and flesh. Cut two wedges and peel them. Chop into chunks and set aside. Reserve the rest of the cantaloupe in a refrigerator.

Wash the celery and cut into small pieces. Set aside.

Wash the basil thoroughly under cold running water. Drain and torn with hands. Set aside.

Wash the cucumber and cut into thick slices. Set aside.

Now, process avocado, cantaloupe, celery, basil, and cucumber in a juicer. Transfer to serving glasses and refrigerate for 15 minutes before serving.

Enjoy!

Nutritional information per serving: Kcal: 288, Protein: 7.5g, Carbs: 37.1g, Fats: 23g

36. Melon Carrot Juice

Ingredients:

1 large honeydew melon wedge

2 large carrots

1 large artichoke

1 large grapefruit

1 small ginger root knob, 1-inch

2 oz of water

Preparation:

Cut the honeydew melon lengthwise in half. Scoop out the seeds using a spoon. Cut a large wedge and peel it. Cut into small chunks and place in a bowl. Wrap the rest of the melon in a plastic foil and refrigerate.

Wash the carrots and cut into thick slices. Set aside.

Using a sharp knife, trim off the outer wilted layers of artichoke. Cut into small chunks and set aside.

Peel the grapefruit and divide into wedges. Set aside.

Peel the ginger knob and set aside.

Now, process, artichoke, grapefruit, honeydew melon, carrots, and ginger in a juicer.

Transfer to serving glasses and stir in the water. Add some ice and serve immediately.

Enjoy!

Nutritional information per serving: Kcal: 230, Protein: 9.5g, Carbs: 72.6g, Fats: 1.1g

37. Apple Lime Juice

Ingredients:

1 large green apple, cored

1 large lime, peeled

1 cup of mango chunks

1 large orange, peeled

1 small ginger root knob, 1-inch

2 oz of water

Preparation:

Wash the apple and remove the core. Cut into bite-sized pieces and set aside.

Peel the lime and cut lengthwise in half. Set aside.

Wash the mango and cut into chunks. Fill the measuring cup and refrigerate the rest for some other juice.

Peel the orange and divide into wedges. Set aside.

Peel the ginger knob and set aside.

Now, process mango, orange, apple, lime, and ginger in a juicer. Transfer to serving glasses and stir in the water.

Add some ice and serve immediately.

Enjoy!

Nutritional information per serving: Kcal: 268, Protein: 12.8g, Carbs: 53g, Fats: 1.5g

38. Kale Lettuce Juice

Ingredients:

1 cup of kale, torn

1 cup Romaine lettuce, torn

1 cup of crookneck squash

1 cup of collard greens, torn

1 large cucumber

½ tsp of Himalayan salt

¼ tsp of Cayenne pepper, ground

2 oz of water

Preparation:

Combine collard greens, kale, and lettuce in a colander. Wash thoroughly under cold running water and torn with hands. Set aside.

Wash the crookneck squash and cut in half. Scoop out the seeds using a spoon. Cut into small chunks and set aside. Reserve the rest for another juice.

Wash the cucumber and chop into thick slices. Set aside.

Now, combine crookneck squash, collard greens, kale, lettuce, and cucumber ina juicer and process until juiced.

Transfer to serving glasses and stir in the salt, Cayenne pepper, and water. Refrigerate for 15 minutes before serving.

Nutritional information per serving: Kcal: 91, Protein: 7.8g, Carbs: 25.2g, Fats: 1.6g

ADDITIONAL TITLES FROM THIS AUTHOR

70 Effective Meal Recipes to Prevent and Solve Being Overweight: Burn Fat Fast by Using Proper Dieting and Smart Nutrition

By

Joe Correa CSN

48 Acne Solving Meal Recipes: The Fast and Natural Path to Fixing Your Acne Problems in Less Than 10 Days!

By

Joe Correa CSN

41 Alzheimer's Preventing Meal Recipes: Reduce or Eliminate Your Alzheimer's Condition in 30 Days or Less!

By

Joe Correa CSN

70 Effective Breast Cancer Meal Recipes: Prevent and Fight Breast Cancer with Smart Nutrition and Powerful Foods

By

Joe Correa CSN

CPSIA information can be obtained
at www.ICGtesting.com
Printed in the USA
BVHW010829250619
551906BV00011B/73/P